44 Things Parents Should Know About Healthy Cooking For Kids

To Tamara, Leah, Elijah, and Jaiden. I *am* and this
book *is* and *because*
you *are*. With peace and love, I dedicate this to you.

44 Things Parents Should Know About Healthy Cooking For Kids

Chef Rock Harper

TURNER

PUBLISHING COMPANY

4507 Charlotte Avenue, Suite 100
Nashville, TN 37209
Phone: (615) 255-2665

www.turnerpublishing.com

44 Things Parents Should Know About Healthy Cooking For Kids

ISBN: 978-1-59652-744-7 (pbk)

Printed in the United States of America

10 11 12 13 14 15 16 17—0 9 8 7 6 5 4 3 2 1

In America, a parent puts food in front of a child
and says, "Eat it, it's good for you."
In Europe, the parent says, "Eat it. It's good!"

~ *John Levee,*
Another Way of Living: A Gallery of Americans
Who Choose to Live in Europe *by John Bainbridge*

Contents

Introduction

Introduction

Everybody's doing it. Every television station and every magazine you flip through, you can't help but see the evidence of someone talking about living a healthy lifestyle or promoting sustainability. Healthy eating has reached or is on the verge of a "tipping point," to borrow the phrase from Malcom Gladwell.

When we see celebrities doing something, we generally want to do it also. However, we, the regular people of the world, need help doing it. If Jay-Z has a watch that I covet, chances are after a few minutes on the Internet I can figure out what kind it is. If not, I'll just call my young nephew Rick, and I'm in good shape. When Sarah Jessica Parker shows up in heels that make women's jaws drop, chances are that you can find out how to get them. When Jamie Oliver has a reality show that tells you that your kids are dying eating the food you and their schools feed them, where do you go to get the good stuff? Ebay or GQ can't help you on this one.

You are left to tons of advice from tons of "experts" on eating healthy. I don't claim to be a nutrition expert, but these 44 Things can help you on your journey. Too many times we are given instructions on healthy eating that don't address specific concerns. You won't find that here. Having trouble introducing new foods to your kid? The chapter "iPod, blindfold, and a spoon" may be the Thing for you. If your kid eats one or more meals at school, I suggest you read "Remember, breakfast pizza is okay to these people."

Yes, I am a chef. But this book isn't loaded with recipes, and I don't think you need them. As a matter of fact, I know you don't. I have tons of cookbooks, and none of them gives you specific instructions or the actual "how-to" when it comes to making a change towards healthy cooking. *44 Things* will do just that—give you the "how-to." If you're looking for recipes, we can pull those up on our phones while shopping in the store!

Use this book as guide for now and years to come. You may take one Thing and have that be your focus for months. That's okay. "Success is achieved by those who are always willing to take the next step, whatever that step may be." Beautiful words from Ralph Marston to keep you encouraged while you change for you and your kids.

As you embark on this new journey, you will come across an enormous amount of information. Keep this Julia Child quote close to your heart; it always helps me: "In spite of food fads, fitness programs, and health concerns, we must never lose sight of a beautifully conceived meal."

The 44 Things

~ 1 ~
Skip commercials

~ 1 ~
Skip commercials

So, I may kill a couple of my endorsement deals on this one, but who cares?

I was sitting in my living room last night with my family watching *Martin,* when this woman just burst into my house and began rapping about how excited she was when she purchased her $1 breakfast sandwich from McDonald's! This woman was young, attractive, and very fashionable, someone my daughter might want to resemble when she gets older. A couple of other people in her entourage were rapping also. As you can probably guess, they were pretty good-looking people too. I imagine they knew I was watching a program laden with an African-American cast and figured I had an affinity for rap music, which would help convince me to buy the garbage she was selling.

Well, I just sat there in disgust as they totally interrupted my family time with something I wasn't in the market for. I wasn't buying it, and they left a few seconds later. But they didn't leave without giving me the impression that they would return. The female rapper showed me an image of her company logo that read underneath "Billions and Billions served," and followed the nifty rap with a jingle that went a little something like "ba da ba ba ba . . . I'm lovin' it!" That darn jingle was stuck in my head, and my kids were singing it. She had to be stopped, and I had to get her from getting to my kids. So I switched over to the Science Channel to watch *How It's Made,* and just when we thought we had found our refuge, she was back in my living room! Only this time she had a different pitch with animals, a different song, and different people.

Some of these companies use my favorite celebrities and my kids' favorite animated creatures—cunning little tricks to try to get my family to buy garbage. I mean, this is my living room, in my house! How dare they? I called the cops and asked if they could get the intruders out of my house. They laughed for about thirty seconds straight before hanging up on me. I did get some good advice through the laughter though: "Just mute the television, idiot!" I totally agree with that statement—well, except for the idiot part, of course.

I hope you can see what I'm getting at. I hate commercials. I am even known to turn to a channel when a program comes on, pause the show for about ten minutes, and then come back to watch it so I have some fast-forward buffer room. This really annoys my family, but cheap, corny, obvious attempts to get my family to purchase crap that I am not asking for really, *really* annoys me too.

What does this have to do with nutrition? The big boys that are selling the horrible food have many tricks up their sleeves. You couldn't begin to imagine the research that goes into making a commercial, let alone the millions and millions of dollars spent to get your family to buy garbage. In an hour-long TV show, about twenty minutes can be for advertising. That's almost half of the actual show! How much time do you have to spend trying to convince your kid that drinking Coca-Cola every day isn't cool? If you gave me twenty minutes of every hour to sell you and your kids something, I could make you buy your own car from me, especially if I hired Beyonce, Miley Cyrus, Michael Jordan, and Justin Bieber. When is the last time you saw your child's favorite celebrity eating kale, broccoli, apples, and quinoa?

We as parents fight this fight, and we have to control what is within our world, which is at home. It's hard to fight these people—the stuff on TV looks good! Of course your kids are going to hear about junk and will have many opportunities to purchase it. That's life. But we must empower them with the tools and knowledge to make the right decisions when they "fly solo." Skipping or muting commercials is a small part of the equation, but trust me, it helps. Skipping commercials is a great time to have a quick discussion about what you've just watched and engage your child in meaningful conversation. Two minutes is a ton of time to ask what your family thinks about the story line so far. What's the end going to be? Who is your favorite so far? What would you have done differently?

I want to buy what I want to buy and when I want to buy it. I assume that you are the same—you didn't get this book because you were suckered into getting it. You bought it because you want you and your family to have a healthy life.

So the next time some pretty lady barges into your living room serenading her way into your child's arteries, politely escort her out.

~ 2 ~
Eat in full meals as opposed to entrees only

− 2 −
Eat in full meals as opposed to entrees only

How many of our meals consist of a meat, starch, and possibly a vegetable? I would imagine a lot. Chicken, rice, and peas. Meatloaf, mashed potatoes, and green beans. Fish sticks, tater tots, and ketchup. Yeah, ketchup is the vegetable; I don't make this up, people—I only write what I see. Any of these sound familiar? Of course they do, it's the American way! It's how I grew up, and more than likely how we feed our children every day. There is nothing wrong with it; I just believe that there are too many missed opportunities to eat better when we feed our families this way. I think a meal should be treated like a sweet song or a beautiful story; this is how we construct meals in a restaurant. Come with me in my world for a moment.

First, a chef will serve something to "wake" the palate up and stimulate the appetite, something we call an aperitif—maybe a glass of dry champagne served with some cheese, fruit, and crackers. This course may be served standing up at the opening cocktail reception. At many nice restaurants, you might have a treat from the chef, like a bite of something very tasty and small. This course is often referred to as an amuse-bouche; again, we are trying to excite this appetite and ready it for what is to come. Also, these little bites can go a long way to satisfy your guests' appetites throughout the entire meal. By the end of the meal, they shouldn't be hungry. After the chef's treat, there can be many different directions in which the meal can go. As a guest, I have eaten over twenty courses at some places; in other places, I go straight to the entrée. You may finish with a dessert course, cheese, and an after-dinner drink.

Sounds pretty easy to create at home, right?

Okay, that was a joke. Well, sort of. Either way,

refrain from throwing the book away and cursing my name. Keep reading.

What does this have to do with my family eating healthy, you ask? Great question! Here's the answer.

It's much harder for children to eat all of the healthy things they need in one meal than it is with several "courses." One of the *Things* I write about is taking a weekly tally of what your children are eating and for them to share this experience. This practice helps us look at the big picture. Couple that with feeding our children at multiple times throughout the day (courses for us), we can capitalize on that same principle.

We generally eat breakfast, lunch, and dinner—three meals—each day. Many children in this country eat half or more of their meals at school. So use your time with them as courses, as opposed to trying to plop one meal in front of them and get all the nutrition on one plate. Try having an aperitif and amuse-bouche waiting for them when they get home at 4:00 P.M. Trade the champagne and aged parmesan for some fresh juice or refreshing water served alongside a small plate of treats. Maybe a quarter of an apple, a few grapes, a couple pieces of cheese, yogurt, raisins, wheat tortilla wraps, carrot sticks, marinated green beans, tomato and cheese with a little olive oil on crackers—the possibilities are endless! They can munch on this while doing homework.

Just before dinner we can get right into course one. How about a salad or a soup? Easy does it, something chopped, quick, flavorful, and small. You don't want it to be too big—remember, they had a small treat, and you will have more nutrition in the entrée. Course one provides the family with more healthy food in small portions, and it also relieves the pressure of making so much food for just the main entrée, where we tend to overeat the wrong things. Make sure you serve bread with the meal, something healthy like a wheat roll.

Last of all, finish with something sweet and small. Make sure you have this prepared in advance, so it doesn't take you away from the table too much. Just last night I bought puff pastry dough, cut it, sprinkled it with a touch of cinnamon sugar, and then baked it. I finished it with fresh fruit, and it was a nice healthy treat that the family enjoyed. Sure puff pastry has fat in it, but remember, we aren't scared of fat—we should consume it responsibly. You shouldn't be afraid either!

Start small, and soon enough, you, too, will be making twenty-course meals!

— 3 —
Enjoy a healthy breakfast

– 3 –

Enjoy a healthy breakfast

"It takes some skill to spoil a breakfast—even the English can't do it."
                                    –John Kenneth Galbraith

I will say this once and only once, so pay attention: Eggs came second. If eggs came before the chicken, we would have eaten them, sending the chicken's existence into oblivion.

And with eggs, we think breakfast.

Breakfast is said to be the most important meal of the day, and for good reason! It is our first shot at getting our fuel for the day ahead. Why do you see so many people drinking energy drinks at 10 A.M. at work? Because they didn't put the right "gas in their tanks." When was the last time you went to the service station and asked for twelve gallons of water to fill your tank? Never, I hope, or you're probably reading this on the bus. Either way, you put the stuff in your tank that makes your car go. Same thing for our kids—we need to "fuel" them with good energy in the morning, the best way to give them the opportunity to have a great day. Doughnuts are not breakfast. Toast with butter and jelly is not breakfast. Waffles with syrup is not breakfast. Frozen pastries filled with "fruit" and topped with icing are not breakfast; it doesn't matter what the box says. Our bodies need food that will give us energy and help us maintain focus until lunch or the next snack.

You wonder why your kid or others are not focused in class? Try taking a look at what they eat. If they eat in the cafeteria, get them out of there! Many schools serve absolute garbage for breakfast, like sausage pizza, so check out the menu before you send them to eat. If they eat at home, great! We can control how energized and focused they will be with the food we serve.

Whole grains at breakfast are needed in a big

way. Toast and waffles aren't bad at all, they just shouldn't stand alone. Sugar is the biggest killer at breakfast, and I mean killer literally. We are killing our families with too much of the wrong kind of sweets. Waffles need syrup, I get it. Heat the syrup up; cold syrup takes more to cover your waffle. Use lite syrup, or make your own with alternative sweeteners (very cheap and easy). Add fruit to them too!

Our desire for sweet stuff isn't bad, it's just the bad sweet stuff we usually use to satisfy that craving. Use fresh fruits—they are full of sweetness! I make applesauce from scratch, and it's so easy I can give you the recipe right here.

- 3 pounds apples, peeled and cored
- 4 strips of lemon peel and the juice
- 1 teaspoon cinnamon
- Pinch of salt
- 1/4 cup raw sugar
- 1 cup of water

Put all of this in a pot with a lid and simmer for thirty minutes, then remove the lemon peel. Mash and blend, or run through a food processor and enjoy.

Having trouble getting the kids to eat fruit? Leave the fruit out on the counter in the morning; it tastes better at room temperature.

Low-fat dairy is helpful for a healthy breakfast. Mix some 2% milk with a great whole-grain cereal and toss in some fruit, and you're in great shape.

I could write an entire book on eggs—I absolutely love them. Eggs are one of the best sources of protein available. I know that people write about the high levels of cholesterol and fat. I'm not a doctor or a nutritionist, so I won't make any claims against them, but we eat them just about every day. I do buy carton egg whites and mix them in with the scramble to give me more protein without the fat. Boiled, poached, baked, scrambled, fried in a bit of olive oil, deviled, or any other way, eggs are fabulous! And best of all, they are cheap.

Begin your day with eggs, or any lean protein supplemented with whole grains, low-fat dairy, and fresh fruit.

— 4 —

Move your butt!

— 4 —

Move your butt!

I will start by sharing a quote from my wonderful wife Tamara, said while we were watching a swimsuit fashion show the other day:

"She looks great, I hate her!"

Sound familiar? I'm sure that line got a chuckle from you; either you've said it or have heard a woman say it before. Tamara doesn't actually hate them, and neither do you—it's a slight-handed compliment, really. She and I often have heated discussions about how and why the women came to have great bodies; she contends that celebrities have help in ways that we regular people can't imagine. I say that isn't always accurate. I don't care if Halle Berry has a personal trainer for every body part, a chef for each day of the week, and a doctor on hand to check

22

her health; she still has to get up and move her butt, as Gordon Ramsay says (but with expletives)!

When you live an active lifestyle, you will *want* to eat better, and so will your kids. Eat a bag of chips, drink a soda, and follow that up with some cookies and ice cream, then try to play a game of catch with your child. (By the way, your Wii doesn't count.) Yeah, let me know how it goes after you wake up from your nap. It's not like this reaction is a revelation from up above. Every time we visit the Killer Clown and scarf down his burgers, nuggets, and shakes, we feel like crap. Even if we do some physical activity afterward, our bodies don't get the benefit they otherwise would because they are full of trash.

My family has been changing while I've been writing this book, and I can see the change in my children. When we eat healthy in the morning, they have awesome results at school. When we are active, our bodies crave the flavorful stuff it really needs. Your body wants the good stuff to be active all day;

you just have to train it, or reprogram it.

So get up! Move that bottom and listen to your body afterward. Does it say "feed me death in a box"? I think not.

– 5 –
Ciao down!

– 5 –
Ciao down!

I have yet to travel to a city that doesn't have some form of Italian food. In Georgia, where pecans and peaches are king, you will find it easy to locate pizza and pasta. Travel to Milwaukee and have yourself a traditional fish fry on Friday, and you will pass a few Italian spots before Saturday. Of course, in New York and Chicago you will find a ton of Italian food, but I have even seen Italian eats in Springfield, Missouri, a quiet, rural city that has some great people and a Bass Pro Shop the size of Bermuda. Speaking of Bermuda, it, too, has a number of Italian restaurants, way more than you would think for an island off the coast of Carolina.

I believe this is so because we the people have decided that Italian is our collective comfort food.

Don't write me off just yet; look around you first. Even though we Americans have a skewed view of what true Italian food is, it's still everywhere you go. I say you should use the love of this fabulous cuisine to cook healthy for your children.

Pizza may come to mind first when you think Italian. Just about everyone loves pizza, and your kids will love eating this homemade pie. Making pizza healthy is as easy as using whole-wheat flour for the crust, low-fat cheese, fresh tomatoes instead of sauce, turkey pepperoni instead of pork, and adding your child's favorite vegetables. If you don't have time for all of that, whole-wheat tortillas and canned crushed tomatoes is a great alternative. Make sure you don't pack on the cheese either; great pizza doesn't need extra cheese.

Pasta is synonymous with the red, white, and green also. I don't believe that enough paper exists to list all of the healthy possibilities with pasta. Start by using whole wheat pasta; there should be a few varieties at your grocery store. Even if you don't use whole wheat pasta, you can add just about anything you want to your family's favorite pasta dish. Broccoli and plum tomatoes, onions paired with zucchini, spinach and chickpeas—the possibilities are endless. But try not to overload on the unhealthy add-ins. Sure, grated cheese is a must on most pasta dishes. But if you cover your healthy pasta in a snowstorm of formaggio, you will have wasted much of your effort.

I absolutely love Italian food, and it encompasses much more than pizza and pasta. I believe that it is the "freshest" of all cuisines. You have to use fresh, whole foods to make great Italian food—not expensive, just fresh and wholesome. It's hard to make awesome Italian eats by using crappy ingredients.

Much of what many Americans have come to know about Italian food has been modified by, well, us Americans. We have a way of changing things around here to fit us and our tastes. So do some research on the different types of Italian cooking before you rush out to try what we have learned to make by eating at Olive Garden.

One Italian chef I worked with used to get a daily request for pasta with "Alfredo sauce." His response to the guests: "Who is this Alfredo you speak of? I don't know him."

Cook with love and Italian flavors, and your children will be constantly asking you for more healthy food. Your response when dinner is ready: *Mangia! Mangia!*

– 6 –

Take a toll at the
end of the week

— 6 —

Take a toll at the end of the week

Food pyramids, calorie counts, BMIs, blah-blah-blahs and some more yaddy-yaddy-yaddas. Eating healthy can be a seemingly tough task if you listen to all of the experts out there. Don't get me wrong, I do not hate on the tools that are available. They can be extremely useful. However, I would be kidding if I suggested that they were easy to follow, though. This book and the tools that I write about may be a little overwhelming to some; I know it's tough for me to employ them with my kids. But it is surely worth it when I look back at the changes we have steadily made over months and months of keeping at it. But getting there starts with one step. One change for you and your children can be the difference. Don't beat yourself or your kids up about not having the perfect meals two weeks after starting better eating habits. It takes time, and you have to track your progress. Celebrate the smallest of changes, for you and the young ones!

I was fortunate enough to meet a family in Philadelphia last year, and we spoke of ways to get kids to eat healthy. The mom gave me an awesome idea: take a toll at the end of the week and praise the weekly success!

This makes total sense to me for a number of reasons. I hate to pressure my kids, but I want them to be aware of the choices that they make on a daily basis. So we do speak with them about food and drink all the time. Sometimes Elijah will eat fruit at school or have chocolate milk with his lunch, while other times he will come home only to have eaten pizza and chips. As upset as that makes me and as much as I want to get on to him about it, I don't want to scare him into not telling me the truth. I also don't want him to grow up a food snob; cafeteria pizza was one of the things that kept me in school!

So, we encourage him to make better choices at school. An apple on Monday, carrots on Wednesday, and grapes on Thursday combined with what they eat at home can begin to look pretty good at the end of the week. You will begin to see how well your kids do and where they need to improve.

The tally of healthy foods eaten each day can be typed on the computer or written. However you do it, take the toll at the dinner table on Saturday night. This is a great conversation piece and another way to get the kids excited about and involved in the daily decisions they make.

Whether you use just one Thing out of this book or employ all 44, keep track of your progress, and give yourself a pat on the back for even picking it up.

— 7 —
The "d" word

– 7 –
The "d" word

1. a : food and drink regularly provided or consumed b : habitual nourishment c : the kind and
amount of food prescribed for a person or animal for
a special reason d : a regimen of eating and drinking
sparingly so as to reduce one's weight.

According to *Merriam-Webster's Collegiate Dic-tionary* (11th ed.), that is the definition of what
I call the "d" word.

I'm sure you already know what the "d" word is,
but just in case you don't, I will reluctantly write it.
Diet.

How many thoughts went through your head
when you just read the "d" word? What were they
about? Did you have a quick daydream about the
number of salads you've eaten over the years? Or

did you begin to count how many of the "d" words you have been on after hearing about your favorite celebrity losing thirty pounds in thirty days on the same "d" word?

To begin to cook healthy for your family, you must first get rid of the unhealthy stuff. In the United States, the manner in which we have been conditioned to think of what the "d" word means is unhealthy. In my experience, the "d" word is used as a temporary fix to achieve a weight-loss goal. Either that or your doctor says you have to go on a "d" word. Whatever the case may be, we don't see "d" words as something we will adapt to our lives and maintain for years to come.

So if you care about your children's eating habits, never, *ever* use the dirty "d" word! When you associate healthy eating with the "d" word, children are conditioned to think of it as something temporary. Not to mention the first three letters of the "d" word spell out what we are trying to avoid happening as long as possible. Right? I eat better than I did before because I want to live and I want my family with me!

Society teaches us that "d" words are very hard and only worth the work if you want to look good for the beach next month, fit into that dress for the wedding, or achieve some other short-term goal. When you introduce some or all of the steps that you are reading about to your children, call it the "new lifestyle for our family," "our food for life," or something that is clever and fun. Use a title that your family will respond to. Whatever you do, refrain from using the "d" word. If you call your new habits a "d" word, they will soon end because all "d" words end sooner or later. Your children will follow suit and will constantly wonder when this whole "d" word thing will be over already.

Of course, there are exceptions to the rule, as always. There are times in our lives when we need to go on the "d" word. Use it responsibly or as directed, and go back to your new and improved eating lifestyle. The better you and your kid feed yourselves, the less likely you will need the "d" words anyway.

When you adopt healthy eating habits, they will be a foundation for the future, and you must do everything in your power to maintain them. Sure, you will have some setbacks—you're human! But don't look at it as a temporary thing. It will be a new and exciting part of your family's life. Remember: life for you, death for the "d" word.

— 8 —
iPod, blindfold, and a spoon

– 8 –
iPod, blindfold, and a spoon

As many of you may know, I was fortunate enough to be a contestant on a reality show a couple of years ago, and I won. I could write an entire book on my experience on *Hell's Kitchen,* but I will share something with you from the show that will help you cook healthier for your children. (Don't worry, you don't have to curse at your children or shout "You donkey!" to pull this one off.)

People call *Hell's Kitchen* host Gordon Ramsay many names, like [expletive], [expletive], [expletive], and I once heard someone say he was worse than six [expletives]! As you can see, I won't dare write most of them in this family-friendly book. All joking aside, I love the man. He is a phenomenal soul with an inspiring energy. I would call him an awesome teacher. I learned a great deal from him, and I believe you can too!

On the show, there is a challenge in which contestants taste foods and have to identify them. Sounds pretty easy, right? Well, throw in blindfolds, headphones with music blaring in your ears, and an English chef with a mean streak, and it can get pretty tough. The goal of the exercise is for us to truly taste our food and to develop that little thing we call a palate. We are artists, and the more "colors" we have on our palates, the better equipped we will be to have awesome careers. I don't want to go all "foodie" on you, but it's an awesome test that you can try at home. Even though many of you may not be training little "Chef Rocks" or "Rockettes," this will make it fun for anyone you are trying to introduce new flavors to. Sure, your kids don't have a famous chef and an audience of ten million people to add to the pressure, but the goal is to have the kids learn, not make them have nightmares.

All you need are about eight to ten food items,

something to cover their eyes with (no dirty socks, please; that's just cruel), and music playing on headphones. The ingredients don't have to be exotic; you want your kids to have fun with healthy food that they have tasted before. Carrots, egg whites, spinach, scallops, arugula, potatoes, apples, rice, herbs, and blueberries are all easy to use—the possibilities are endless! Cook them with no seasoning (food blasphemy, except here) so they are able to taste only the food. Mash it up so they can't easily identify what it is from its texture.

We have five senses, and it is said that when you take away one or more, it enhances the remaining ones. So with the music, we are trying to focus on taste only here. Don't forget that the eyes send a message to the brain when it sees a food. Take spinach, for instance. The brain may tell us that we hate spinach because it's nasty. More times than not, we believe our brains, especially when we are kids. By the time we get around to tasting the spinach, we reject it before we even swallow. Well, using a blindfold takes away the prejudice and allows the taster to focus on just the flavor. They still may not like it, but the taste will be stored in their memory for future reference. I believe the more foods and flavors our children are familiar with, the more apt they will be to try new foods. Many of us have this notion that healthy food is limited and lacks flavor, when the truth is exactly the opposite.

You can introduce new foods like this; just make it a bonus round or something. So when you cook the new food in the future, your children may not be so reluctant to try.

Just as I have a goal of becoming a better chef, that wasn't the only reason I went on *Hell's Kitchen;* I made a little bit of money too. Let's be real, the promise of being a conscious little eater may not be appealing to your young ones. They may tell you like Smokey told his mother in the film *Friday,* "This ain't enough!" So we have to sweeten the pot a bit. Money always works, of course, but just make it reasonable. Maybe the winner can pick dinner or dessert one day next week; just make sure you give them the choice of their favorites. If you have an only child, they can compete against their own score.

Unlike in the reality show, remember that it is more important to encourage the kids to try rather than to always win. So you may choose to award prizes to all children (perhaps still making the winner's a bit more desirable than the other prizes). The last thing you want to do is to turn this into a bitter competition and turn them off completely!

So load up your playlists, make sure the blindfolds can't be seen through, and have fun training those healthy little eaters!

– 9 –

Pitch a tent and pack a picnic basket

− 9 −

Pitch a tent and pack a picnic basket

Who doesn't love the great outdoors? Okay, I set myself up on that one, because my wife detests the outdoors. Unless, of course, the outdoors come with an air-conditioned hotel room. But we all love the food that comes with the experience of taking a trip!

If you ever want to figure out a way to incorporate healthy foods into your meals, take a trip—to your living room, that is. I feel like my kids will try new and healthy foods when cuisine has a theme. Take asparagus, for instance. I love them, especially when they're in season. My kids? Maybe not so much. But if we roll out a blanket on the living room floor and have an indoor barbecue, I have already set the stage for excitement, and children are more receptive to new things when creativity and imagination are present. Dim the lights, put on a favorite movie, tell quick stories, and have the food match the theme. A little olive oil, salt, pepper, and lemon juice on those grilled asparagus make them even more approachable in the midst of all of the family fun.

As you have read, I am a big fan of the family eating together at the table. But the table is the table, and it can become a bit redundant after a while. So switch it up and have fun with it! Anywhere you can imagine traveling, do it in your house, and you will find tons of ways to incorporate healthy food. You can even use movies as your guide! How about recreating a dish from a favorite family film? (*Ratatouille,* anyone?)

Remember, the goal is to cook healthier and have a great time doing it. I believe that eating should be a fun and memorable experience. Enjoyable food doesn't have to be far away or expensive—find it, and bring it to the family.

— 10 —
Stouffer's has it half right

– 10 –
Stouffer's has it half right

I hope I don't get in trouble for this chapter, but those who know me know I have to speak the truth the way I see it.

Did you see the "Let's fix dinner" commercial from Stouffer's? As much as I don't like commercials, this one had me at hello. It talks about getting back to the dinner table, connecting with family, and using meals to bring us closer. It's like they stole a copy of my book and made an ad campaign out of it! I know that's what you were thinking, but I have to say that isn't true; it just isn't possible, and I will tell you why in just a little bit.

I know with absolute certainty that the dinner table is and can be a "fixer" for many of our family obstacles. We have to get back to the table, ladies and gentlemen. I don't want to sound too much like the old guy, but we have a disconnect in this beautiful nation that is getting larger by the day. I love my country; I love what the technology here has done for us and will continue to do. But I just don't think parents should have to look on Facebook to find out how their kid's day was. If we take a little time to break bread together, we can tackle some of the stuff we so often say that "we just don't have time for."

One of the biggest issues we as parents face is what our families eat. The more contact we have with the kids, the more we can influence better eating habits. When we get them to sit and have a meal, we have to give them great choices. Children are extremely intelligent these days, and they soak up what they have learned about these good choices, eventually going on to make conscious decisions about their health. Which brings me back to my main point: Stouffer's has it half right—get to the table with your family. The other half is most important, though: feed them healthy food. I think

Stouffer's can't begin to speak on that because of the very nature of the product they sell. I don't want to come off as a food snob, because I'm not. But I know we also need to get away from boxed, frozen, processed garbage disguised as healthy food. Yes, making food does take time, and the frozen stuff is quick and convenient. Well, if you really thought these packaged foods were the key, I honestly don't believe you would be reading this book. You have the desire to change your family, so make the jump.

Get your family to the table and feed them food that will help them live. It isn't hard; it just takes commitment and time. You will be pleasantly surprised (most of the time) about what you will learn from your little ones while sitting at the table eating good food. Most of all, you will be happy that you have your beautiful family together.

When is the last time you held hands with your family? Do you keep asking yourself what your kids like? How often do you wonder when and where your children pick up bad manners? You want to teach boys and girls how to respect each other and themselves? The dinner table is your training ground. I know these aren't specific cooking tips, but they are tools that, if employed collectively, will make it easier to get your children to respect themselves and what they fuel their bodies with.

So turn the TV off, and silence all phones. No toys, no books, no music—just the family and good food. It may seem strange at first, but after a while you will look forward to it, and so will they.

~ 11 ~
Mommy, who put this tertiary butylhydroquinone in my chicken?

– 11 –
Mommy, who put this tertiary butylhydroquinone in my chicken?

Where, oh where, do I begin?

That word you just had a "what-the-heck" moment with is better known as TBHQ. It is a preservative, in short. Basically, companies use it to keep certain fats from going rancid in foods they want to sell us. Why is that a problem, you ask? It isn't, I guess—that is, if nausea, vomiting, and possible fainting aren't problems. These are all symptoms that some people say are side effects of consuming TBHQ in excessive quantities.

Your beloved McNuggets have TBHQ in them . . . and so do certain lacquers, varnishes, and resins. I don't know about you, but I don't want to eat anything that's in varnish. I sure as heck don't want to feed it to my children, either!

You only find this stuff out by reading labels and knowing what is in your food. In order to make it a bit easier on your kids' change toward eating healthy, have them read labels of some of the foods they covet. Having a better understanding of what's in food will help us eat to live.

I encourage my kids to read labels all the time. I then ask if they know what a certain ingredient is. If not, we might do a quick search online and see what we are eating. Sometimes it works, especially if they are young. Sometimes—I have to be honest—it has a small or no effect. Children have said to me, "It tastes so good, Chef Rock! I don't care what's in it."

It's sad, but true.

However, don't let that stop you! Keep pressing on, and occasionally encourage your kids to know what goes in their little bodies. Some people can't even begin to believe that the almighty FDA would allow something into stores that could hurt customers. MSG used to be commonplace, remember? Now if you use it, you are shunned by society. The FDA is still cool with it, though.

Imagine your daughter telling you she doesn't care for that brand of cookies because it has too much sugar in it, or because it contains trans fats. Pretty cool, huh? Mine did, and it made me so proud! I'm not bragging like our children are the best eaters in the world, because they aren't, and they give us a very tough time on a daily basis. But at that moment, I felt like all of the preaching to her was worth it, and she was on her way to making great food decisions.

– 12 –
"Frankly, my dear, I don't give a . . . !"

– 12 –
"Frankly, my dear, I don't give a . . . !"

I know it sounds harsh, but relax and read on.

By a show of hands, how many of us have had our children absolutely refuse to eat something? All of you? Okay, class, you may put your hands down now, I'm here to help.

There is no easy way around this. You will have to be firm and not compromise. Of course, I have written about tools and practices that are "deals" you can make with your kids, but none of them should be unhealthy options.

For instance, we rarely tell Elijah or Leah that if they eat their green beans, they can have a fudge sundae with all the fixings. There is nothing wrong with the occasional sundae, but to tie bad foods to eating healthy as a regular reward isn't a smart move.

In short, we cook what we cook in our home, and they eat what we cook. If not, they don't eat. Sounds harsh? Sorry, that's just how it is. Children are extremely intelligent, and they know how to "work the system." My children have spent hours at the table refusing to eat certain foods. Yes, hours. They have even both fallen asleep while staging their protests at the dinner table!

What's a parent to do?

I will tell you what to do: gently lay your child to bed as you would normally. When they wake, guess what's for breakfast? You got it—last night's goodies! Sometimes, we don't have time for a "pre-school protest" in the morning and would hate to send them to school without their needed energy, so we will save the leftovers for afternoon snack or dinner's appetizer. One thing is clear in this house: we will not waste food, and you eat what is served.

Eventually.

Never get mad when your kids refuse to eat. I

know it is frustrating, but it is why they are here. Yes, to frustrate us. At least that's what we did to my mother.

We as parents have to educate ourselves as to what is best for our children, and then we have to stick with what we know is best. The next time you run into a little resistance when trying to feed them healthy eats, don't hesitate to summon your inner Rhett.

— 13 —

"Nobody puts Baby in a corner."

— 13 —
"Nobody puts Baby in a corner."

Vincent Van Gogh was taught that the only colors that exist are black and brown. He never moved to Paris. He never saw the beautiful sun in the south of France that inspired him so.

Sounds crazy, I know. But imagine if it were true. Would he have been able to create what we revere as some of the world's greatest pieces of art?

Maybe, maybe not.

We both know that what I wrote isn't true, and that Van Gogh's work is regarded as some of the best. I am going to guess that he had a huge palette. In other words, he had a ton of colors to choose from.

Chefs are also artists, and we have palettes too. We build flavor combinations based upon the foods that we are familiar with. The more foods we can recognize, the more culinary art we can create. If a chef is familiar with only butter, cream, and spice, then most of his or her dishes will be spicy and drowned in fat.

The same goes for us as consumers. I encourage you to start as young as you can with your children. As soon as they are able to eat solid foods, begin the taste experiments. Don't limit your babies to the canned stuff; be your own baby-food company. Always talk to your doctor before introducing anything new, but after that, just go for it. Asparagus, butternut squash, collard greens, raspberries, blueberries, and hundreds of other foods will make great puree to feed your little one. Don't be afraid of flavor either; season or sweeten the food and get your child used to what good food is supposed to taste like. Expose your children's tongues to true flavor as early as possible, and when they get older, it will be the norm to appreciate what the body truly needs. When our kids taste all of the processed crap at an early age, it becomes the norm, and then we have to break them of the bad habits. If we don't expose our children to the thousands of different flavors in the world, we limit their chances of making great decisions when they get older. We also increase the likelihood of those "dinner-table protests" that happen so frequently now.

I want my children, and yours, to live beautiful and healthy lives. As a father of beautiful children, I am sometimes faced with the decision of whether or not to try something new with my kids. Should I just cook what they like with no resistance and leave them boxed in for now and the future? I remember what Johnny Castle, played by the late, great Patrick Swayze, said: "Nobody puts Baby in a corner." I encourage you to do the same and not keep your kids in a corner with the same food.

– 14 –
Greasy food bad, fried food good

– 14 –

Greasy food bad, fried food good

Yes, you read correctly. I am writing a book about cooking healthy for your children, and I am here to tell you fried food isn't the devil. If I may borrow a phrase from the eloquent and ever-insightful Ricky Bobby, "That. Just. Happened."

Too often, fried food gets such a bad rap, and with good cause. There are far too many fried-food phonies in this country giving us garbage disguised as true fried food. I don't need to call anyone out in this chapter; just take some guesses. Deep frying may be the best cooking method of all the phonies. Just think about it for a second. What can't you submerge in hot, flavorful fat and not have it come out beautifully? Not too many things. I'm getting hungry just thinking of it! I bet you are too.

What in the world does this have to do with healthy cooking, you ask? As you know, I believe in indulging in "the good stuff" every now and then. I can't subscribe to the school of thought that says not to ever eat fried foods. Nor do I believe for a second that fried chicken submerged in lard should be consumed a couple of times a week. I don't care what age your grandmother lived to, or if she was or is an exception to the rule; God bless her heart (literally). My point is to encourage you to indulge and treat your family to food that has flavor and is cooked properly. You don't need enormous amounts of saturated fat on a daily basis to make your meals taste great. But having them responsibly will make your family appreciate all types of foods. It will also prevent your kids from being the ones who go to school or anywhere away from the house and over-eat garbage food.

Fried food should not be greasy. I know many of you say that's impossible, and I say you are sadly mistaken. Greasy food is literally saturated and soaked in grease. Fried food is moist, full of flavor, and free of excess oil, if done properly.

There are a few things to keep in mind when you fry. The oil has to be able to withstand high temperatures for a long time; these are oils that have a "high smoke point." The wrong fat can break down easily, and it will cook your food improperly and possibly make it greasy. If you cook the food on a low temperature, it will slowly cook and become greasy. Make sure the temperature is high enough, and don't overcrowd your pan to prevent lowering the temperature too fast. Never use old grease. It has broken down and has lost of all of its ability to produce a great fried piece of food. I know Grandma had the can of grease on the back of her stove for your entire childhood. You aren't her—she had a gift, and I'm here to tell you that sadly, you don't have her gift yet. Besides, she never really used that grease; it was just a great cover-up for her hidden stash of fresh peanut oil in the pantry. Clean your oil, and store it away from light and air when not in use. After all, we aren't going to use this oil that much. Lastly, drain your food in a single layer on a rack or drain pan of some sort; towels just soak back into the food.

So I kind of went a little off course in this chapter just to make the point that we should never be afraid to have a treat every now and then. If you are a calorie counter, that's cool—count them, and then get back on track after you finish. When you do decide to dive in, just make sure it isn't out of control, and be certain your family enjoys the good stuff the way it should be eaten.

— 15 —

"Be the change you want
to see in the world."

– 15 –

"Be the change you want to see in the world."

I won't beat around the bush with this one. For the sake of the topic, your "world" in this piece of advice from Gandhi is your household.

If you are reading this while sucking down your 1,000 calorie moofoolatte, check yourself. You have to change you before you change anything for your children. I know you're the parent and you do what you want. I know you work harder than they do and deserve a little treat. I am aware of so many of the excuses that you keep in your pocket to justify your unhealthy addictions because I used to use them! My wife and I have had many "discussions" on this very topic. Tamara is of the mindset that she is an adult and can make her own decisions responsibly. Well, what can we honestly say to our children when they see us eating and drinking garbage and they want a bite or a sip? "No, you can't destroy your body, but I can destroy mine, because I'm an adult." Do as I say, not as I do doesn't work, my friends. Our children will resent us for it. Yes, we are still talking about eating healthy food.

I recently talked to my children about getting off the couch and away from the television and Internet. They said, "Okay, can you come outside with us, Daddy?" When I responded with my usual "I'm too tired, I work really hard, blah, blah, blah," I could tell it was disappointing to them, and it was also hypocritical. How can I expect them to live an active lifestyle if I don't? So we changed. Little by little, I started with myself.

I can't judge anyone; I'm just offering advice that I think will help you out at home. My life is far from perfect, but we are working on us. I implore you to do the same. We don't have time to beat around the bush with excuses and behavior that keeps the problems alive and kicking. We have to break away immediately! Some people say to throw out all the garbage food in your house and start fresh today. I will echo that only if you can afford to do so. Most of us can't, so I encourage you to slowly get rid of the junk. Incorporate new healthy food until all the garbage is gone. Any start is better than no start at all. It is going to be tough, but we must start with us. Otherwise, we will look like dictators (even though to them, we probably already do).

If you do maintain a separate set of rules for yourself, when your kids are able to get out and make their own decisions, they will repeat your behavior, and the cycle will continue. To make eating healthy the norm, you should go above and beyond what they do.

If this is going to work, you have to take a long, hard look in the mirror and decide what your future is going to look like. Not just for the example you are setting for the children, but for your own personal health. You have a beautiful family, and you can't be around for them if you constantly load your body with crap. You possess the desire to change, or else you wouldn't bother to read this. It doesn't have to be all about lettuce and rice crackers—the day of that thinking has come and gone. Eating healthy can be fun, flavorful, and such a great start to a fruitful future.

Gandhi also said, "Men often become what they believe themselves to be. If I believe I cannot do something, it makes me incapable of doing it. But when I believe I can, then I acquire the ability to do it even if I didn't have it in the beginning." I think you believe you can do this. I would surely have to agree.

– 16 –
Put another bun in the oven!

~ 16 ~

Put another bun in the oven!

Why would you gasp like that? "Putting a bun in the oven" is a common phrase in our culture that means to have a baby? Well, I'm talking about bread and baked goods, people!

People love bread, and so do your children, I imagine. If they have had good bread, chances are they love it. Bread gets a bad rap, and I think it's totally unfair. Especially after some doctor came through years ago and told us that the key to losing weight was to stop eating carbohydrates. What did we do? We stopped eating bread—in front of people, at least.

Bread is a great and affordable source of nutrition and flavor. You can add anything to bread to make it taste great, and even better, it can remain healthy.

Just because I wrote this chapter does not give you license to run out and scarf down four croissants, though. Keep reading, please.

I grew up eating zucchini bread and thinking that my grandmother mistakenly gave me a treat when she thought she was giving me something healthy. There are thousands of recipes available on the Internet that can demonstrate how to bake healthy breads. Some breads can have an extremely high amount of sugar and fat, so find alternatives and use the substitutes. Whole-wheat pastry flour instead of bleached all-purpose flour is one I like to incorporate into my baking. I just purchased some organic blue agave, and it is amazing. It's an all-natural sweetener that is 25 percent sweeter than white sugar, so you use less. Unless you have time and patience to experiment, you should use recipes that have made the substitution already or show you how to change the ingredients. Baking is an exact process, and the slightest change can ruin the entire recipe.

Everyone loves muffins! How about one that is

made with wheat flour, flaxseed, nonfat milk, and a different sweetener? Get a good recipe, and I am sure your family will eat them up! Leah, my seven-year-old daughter, loves to make scones with Daddy, and she just can't wait to eat her finished product. I use whole-wheat flour and evaporated cane sugar along with fruit-juice–sweetened fruit like cranberries, and fat-free buttermilk as alternates to make them healthier. The possibilities are endless.

If you are ever stuck on how to get the kids to eat a healthy treat, remember to "put a bun in the oven!" Bread, of course. Not the other one, unless you want another test subject for this book.

— 17 —

"Why, back in the 30s, children as young as five could work as they pleased; from textile factories to iron smelts. Yippee! Hurray!"

– 17 –

"Why, back in the 30s, children as young as five could work as they pleased; from textile factories to iron smelts. Yippee! Hurray!"

S ome classics (i.e., *Zoolander*) should never die. Why can't kids work? My children perform manual labor all the time! I hope I don't get in trouble for it.

You should make your kids work also. When you take a trip to the store, have them help with the shopping. My family loves to spend money, especially the ladies of my life. Why not use that energy to educate them on healthy choices? My kids love to weigh the produce, and bagging it up always causes an argument. After so many trips to the store, we can send them on healthy scavenger hunts. I have asked my children to find us something high in fiber that we can use for dessert. It is a great feeling when they suggest apples. Hopefully in years to come, they will have a full arsenal of healthy options.

We also read labels in the store while we shop. It's a fun way to keep them busy, which we all know can be tough without blowing a gasket in public. After you have educated them at home on the effects of consuming too much sugar, see if they can pick out a great drink or food by reading the labels. Let them tell you what the bad stuff is too.

Work those math skills also! Show them how much a bag of frozen, processed, salty, fatty fries cost and then show them how much cheaper raw potatoes are. Not only will you show them that healthy food can be cheaper, you will also instill in them a better sense of valuing their money. Do the same for any frozen product or processed product, and you will surprise yourself too! Canned vegetables and fruits are a good example also. The children will be amazed.

I am a believer in rewards, as you know. If the kids do well, get something just for them. But don't reward them with junk; use something that is good for them and tasty. Otherwise, you will be contradicting yourself.

The key is to take some of the pressure that comes with shopping off of yourself while educating your children at the same time.

I urge you, my friends, to listen to Little Cletus! Do not deprive our youth of the right to earn a decent wage. Just keep them away from the textile factories and iron smelts.

— 18 —
Eat out!

− 18 −
Eat out!

Itook my son, Elijah, to the Signature Chefs Auction in Washington, D.C., a few months ago. It is a phenomenal epicurean event where the best chefs in D.C. come together and donate their time and food to help raise money to end premature births.

Let me give you a quick rundown of what he tried that night:

Octopus ceviche with heirloom tomatoes, roasted lamb belly, spinach soufflé, morel mushrooms, roasted beet salad, venison loin cooked medium over micro greens, ricotta gnocchi, and a couple of other things.

The next night at home, he complained about eating his peas.

Give me a break already! I told you I go through

the same madness that you do. We don't raise our kids to be food snobs at all. They respect food and they are extremely humble. But I couldn't for the life of me figure out how my kids would eat these different foods while we were out, but at home it was like they waged a war on the normal stuff. I went as far as to step the ingredients up to see what would happen. I made short-rib ravioli stuffed with a cauliflower puree, chanterelle and morel mushrooms, and black garlic. It was great and I knew they would dive right in. Nope. "Eww, what's that stuff?" I was offended at this point! My ego got hurt because there could be no way these other chefs cook better than me in my own kids' eyes. My wife assured me I could still cook, and I was okay.

It was then we realized that it wasn't my cooking; it was just the fact that it was me, and my wife, for that matter. Our children like going out and trying new things. Just like us, it is exciting for them to dine out and expand their horizons. They will try just about anything while dining out. Some of the stuff I don't even eat, they will.

I used that event as an example, but kids just love going out—it doesn't matter where. Take your kids out and encourage them to try something new. It will help in the future when you cook at home. Realize also that you have to remind them that you are cooking what they had while out; otherwise, it's just something new that you're cooking, and they are programmed to say "yuck." After I reminded Elijah that he had had these mushrooms while we were out, he said, "Oh yeah, I will try that again. That tasted good!"

I'm not making this up, people, it is that simple. Give it a try as often as you can. Just make sure the food is good and the kids have a good time. I think you will be surprised at how open they are to eating new and healthy foods.

— 19 —
Put it in one pot

– 19 –
Put it in one pot

One-pot cookery is amazing for several reasons, most notably, it's amazing.

Many great dishes from around the world are made in a single pot. Macaroni and cheese, chicken potpie, cassoulet, shepherd's pie, paella, jambalaya, osso bucco, risotto—you get the point. I could go on for days.

I am a big fan of beautiful meals that have separate side dishes and accompaniments; it makes the meal more exciting and gives a great opportunity to introduce healthy ingredients. I also am a big fan of practicality. I know that I often find myself short on time, and that's when I cook a meal all in one pot. Many times I don't have the energy or focus to make something elaborate. When we are strapped for time or energy, we normally resort to the frozen stuff or crappy take-out. Even if it's great take-out, it still costs more money and is more than likely not as healthy as a home-cooked meal.

I love the versatility of stews and hearty soups. They are substantial enough to serve as a dinner that will satisfy the whole family, and they often don't cost much. Our children usually enjoy eating one-pot dishes, which makes it easier to add vegetables to. Macaroni and cheese is great, but if you add some broccoli along with whole wheat pasta, it can make the journey towards eating healthy a little easier. Making fried rice? Use brown rice instead of white, switch out the regular soy sauce with the low-sodium alternative, and add Chinese cabbage, snow peas, and any other vegetables that fit.

Never sacrifice flavor; that's why we love the one-pot dishes. Just make sure they're healthy.

– 20 –
Don't be fooled

– 20 –
Don't be fooled

Of course you won't be fooled! You purchased this book and told 5,000 of your closest friends to do the same; I would never take you for a fool. I'm writing this chapter just in case of an emergency.

I saw an ad the other day for a "mango in a bottle," and I was thoroughly bothered. Can you tell by now I don't like commercials? I especially despise the ones that sucker us into buying nonsense, like mangoes in bottles.

Steve White is one of the funniest men I have seen. I was fortunate enough to meet him through some friends in Las Vegas, and he invited us to his show. Tamara and I laughed so much that we may have used two of my asthma inhalers that night—

and she doesn't have asthma, I do. (She was fine, I almost died.)

Steve has a bit in which he talks about the side effects of medicines and processed foods. He tells how he saw a low-calorie sweetener that advertised it contained half the calories of regular sugar, to which he asks the audience, "Do you know what else has half the calories of sugar?" After a moment of no responses, he emphatically replies, "Half the [dang] sugar!"

Back to my original point: when eating and drinking outside of the home, don't be fooled by labels and claims by these companies. We all lead busy lives, and sometimes we have to get food on the go. Some food and drink that appears to be good for us is not. As a matter of fact, they are bad. If you want the nutrients and benefits of a mango, maybe you should eat a mango! I'm just throwing things out there. The actual mango does not have the pre- servatives and processed sugar that are in the bottle.

How many foods on the shelf have we seen that

profess to contain a small amount of calories? "100 calories per serving," they tell us! We jump right away and say, "Wow, that's nothing." Until we realize that the serving is the size of a teaspoon, and by the time we eat as much as an actual human should, we have consumed tons of bad calories.

Just because a product is free from fat doesn't make it healthy. It could be loaded with sugars, and those are just as bad as anything else when consumed improperly.

My kids drink flavored milk at school, and it makes me cringe. I encourage them to drink just plain milk because of all of the junk that is in that pink and brown liquid they call milk.

We have to train our children to be able to taste food and enjoy it without it being masked with all that sugar and salt. Most of the time, we eat these altered foods when we are out of the house and in need of a quick fix. Be aware of what you are actually consuming, and don't be fooled!

— 21 —
Remember, breakfast pizza is okay to these people

– 21 –

Remember, breakfast pizza is okay to these people

Every day, we leave our children with people we barely know, from the school bus driver to the teacher and even the cafeteria employees. I'm talking about our local school systems. We assume that these people must have our children's future and health at the top of their agenda. Most Americans believe we live in the greatest nation in the world; at least I do. How could this great nation allow my child to be exposed daily to hazards but no one speak up? It wouldn't happen, and if it did, someone would surely have to pay, right?

Not so much.

First of all, there is no "Big Brother" watching over every little thing that goes on in this country. That's where the people of this country come into play. We have the right and, some say, the obligation to speak up. This right of ours also pertains to what our children eat at school.

The next time you think there could be no way that your kid would have the option to eat anything terribly unhealthy at school, think again.

I was watching the television program *Jamie Oliver's Food Revolution* on ABC recently. One of the school cafeteria kitchens Jamie was investigating served breakfast pizza, and I was shocked. I was thinking, "Who are these people, and how could they allow that to go on in their school district?" I often try to look in the mirror when I call someone out, so I did just that. I took a look at our children's school menu, and what did I find? Yup! In my own school district in the mighty, mighty Commonwealth of Virginia, breakfast pizza was a healthy option.

I could moan and complain, and so could you. But you have to wake up, and so do I. We have to understand that our kids are wasting all of the effort put in at home if they eat junk at school. Many children eat more than half of their daily food at school. You can cook whatever you like at home, but if they eat crap at school, they will gravitate towards the garbage. Junk foods are like drugs; actually, they are drugs, if you ask me.

I encourage you first to stay active and know what your child is being served each day. We ask our children what they plan to eat every day. We make better decisions as a family. We do have rules, but we allow the kids to be a part of the decision—no one likes to be totally told what to do. When they make mistakes or miss a fruit or a veggie, it is so important that you don't scold them. If a child thinks he is going to get in trouble, he will not tell you the truth the next time. I'm guessing the last thing you want is for your child to be throwing away his fruit and come home and tell you he ate it all.

If you are able to, have them take lunch to school. This way you can control everything, and the kids are really a part of the process. It can be totally personalized to their liking. Be sure to include a treat that they really like. It will serve as a reminder that if one eats well, it's okay to indulge a bit.

Last and maybe most important, get involved. I have an entire Thing dedicated to this subject, but I have to set the stage. We are the customers, and the school systems are our merchants. Know that you are in charge, and use that knowledge to create a better environment for your children. If you think that there isn't a chance that this goes on in your district, check it out, and just remember: breakfast pizza is okay to these people.

— 22 —
You're in a rush, I get it

– 22 –
You're in a rush, I get it

You can probably guess that I am a big fan of getting back to the table and enjoying the family. I think that eating healthy can be a much easier task when we do it together. I also believe that working together as a family can help with so many challenges that we face today. (I could write another book on that subject alone, and I probably will, but that isn't what this Thing is about.)

Plain and simple: we are busier today than we have ever been. Working forty-hour weeks just doesn't exist for most of us. I think it can if we fashion our lives that way, but it doesn't happen as much as it used to. Even if we don't have a full-time job, we still find ourselves wondering what happened to the day that just flew by us.

My wife is a stay-at-home mom, and she often finds herself struggling to get everything done in one day. I'm not even talking about the food yet! We all know how tough it can be to keep a family functional. If you (cough) guys (cough) don't know, I suggest you stay home and manage the house for a few days and get back to me with the results. Like anything else, success in this realm is achievable, but you get there with proper planning and focus.

I do understand that sometimes we are on the run, and making those healthy sit-down meals just may not be in the cards. But there is nothing worse to me than having an awesome "food week" with the family only to have it destroyed by eating fast-food a few times on the weekend. Help is here, my friends. We can eat out and be on the go and still maintain a healthy lifestyle. We just have to know how to make the smart decisions.

The first step is to plan properly. Nothing complicated, just be prepared. Let's say your child has a soccer game on Saturday morning; I am guessing you would know this before Saturday. So make sure you have control of the day before the day actually happens. Plan out breakfast the day prior. Sure, we would love to have the full spread on Saturday morning, but unless you are like my 5 A.M.-rising grandmother, you don't have time for that. A bowl of cereal or oatmeal with fresh fruit, a healthy muffin, nuts, and some of that homemade applesauce you prepared earlier that week are quick and easy options that can help your kids eat healthy on their busy day.

Well, what if you hit the snooze button one time too many? What if it's a little chilly outside? The blankets combined with the warmth of your sweetheart have been known to cause frequent tardiness. At some point, we jump up, and the frenzy begins.

"Hurry up and get ready, we can't be late!" you shout as you think about the conversation you had last week with Jesse's mom. Jesse's mom privately launched a verbal assault on all of the parents who didn't take their constant tardiness seriously, and you agree wholeheartedly. "But I'm hungry," replies the child. Which leads to the favorite motherly response of the fast-food joint: "We will have to grab something quick while we're out!"

And there goes our hard work right out the door. Until now, that is.

First of all, always keep a stash of healthy eats in the pantry. Make sure some of them don't need refrigeration so that you don't need a cooler everywhere you go. Trail mix, dried fruit, nuts, and granola are all snacks you can keep either in the house or in the car just in case of a hunger emergency.

If you must go to the fast-food joints, you have to know how to order. First of all, stay away from the cheese. I know it's good, but it is loaded with garbage and isn't real cheese, by the way—it's processed cheese food. (I have an entire Thing dedicated to this.) So if your choice is to get a breakfast sandwich, try to unload the unhealthy stuff. Get rid of the meat after you take off the cheese. Many times the meat is loaded with fat, water, and other fillers, so when you think you are getting a sausage on a biscuit, you're really not. Skip it and go with an egg sandwich; remember, eggs have great protein. Try to get a poached egg if they offer it, stay away from those fat-laden biscuits, and supplement your meal with other goodies. Many of the fast-food restaurants have added healthier options to the menu after coming under fire by the public, but be careful, because they are loaded with traps too. Crisp apples are a great option; just leave off the candy-like caramel that accompanies them. Yogurts with fruit are showing up on menus and are pretty good options, and even though the fruit isn't fresh, it's better than none at all.

At lunch go for the salads; again, just be careful of the meat, even if it is grilled. More than likely it has been injected with a solution that includes preservatives and extra fat and salt. Many times the dressing that they provide is way too much, so try to use half or less to avoid unnecessary calories.

I use fast-food joints as an example not because

I think we should visit them often. As a matter of fact, I think there are far too many options for us to even patronize many of these places on a regular basis. The fact is that we visit these places because of the way we live. I visit them also; I'm not judging anyone. I know how it is. Sometimes we are out and about, and time flies, and the kids are hungry. What can we tell them? We have to feed them. What's on every corner in most of America? That's right, fast-food garbage. You know that I am all about indulging in the "good stuff" every now and then, but fast-food isn't the "good stuff." There are plenty of restaurants around that offer real, fresh food that was made in an actual kitchen, not some laboratory in another country.

I have lived in the United States my entire life, and that is my only perspective. I totally understand how it is to live here. My vision to have all families back at the table for every meal may not happen this year. I get it. In the meantime, just be smart about your busy-day options, and little by little, you will begin to see progress in your family's eating habits while out and about.

— 23 —

Sorry, sweeties, you have to share me

– 23 –

Sorry, sweeties, you have to share me

Sorry to all of you wannabe players reading this, I'm not in favor of polygamy.

But what are we talking about again? Oh, yes, sharing your sweetie!

Why limit yourself to just one? Most of us have just one and we are told that is okay. My friends, I beg to differ. Variety is the spice of life! Whoever introduced this notion to society that we have to be with the same throughout eternity was a nutcase. I say change it up and have a little fun in your life. It took my wife awhile before she was on board. We didn't really argue about it; she was open to trying new things, but it wasn't easy, though. After a while she came around, and she's glad we started sharing.

Wait a minute. What's wrong with you people?

I'm talking about sugar!

I grew up thinking that white sugar was the primary way to sweeten things. I saw the occasional brown sugar and honey use, but white sugar was king. Over the years I have found out that I can use many other products to sweeten food—many times healthier than white sugar.

Sugar gets a bad rap, and it shouldn't all of the time. As with anything, we must learn to enjoy things in moderation. Too much of anything is bad. (Well, many things, not everything.)

There are a few alternative artificial sweeteners on the market. Equal, Stevia, Sweet 'N Low, Truvia, and Splenda are just a few. I won't go into which ones are better than others, but as with any new product, do your research before using them. Many people have said they have had negative side effects while using these products, but many people love the products too. I have cooked with all of them, and of course I like natural sugars better than these, but they do have their place. I have a few diabetic friends who are amazed when I can offer dessert that they can actually eat. I was fortunate enough to cook extensively with Equal when I was working at B. Smith's. B. Smith was endorsing Equal and created a ton of recipes using the product, and it was my job to execute these dishes for the menu. I wasn't thrilled about the task at first, but in the end, it made me a better chef. I don't use artificial sweeteners enough to give a ringing endorsement, but it may be worth a shot for you and your family.

My newest love is agave nectar. It comes in liquid form and is probably at your grocery store. Agave is much sweeter than sugar, which means you can use less. It also has a desirable low-glycemic index, which means that when consumed, it won't cause a sharp rise or fall in blood sugar. One cup of sugar is equal to one-third cup of agave in sweetness. I cook and bake with it—this stuff is amazing. (Just don't replace sugar in recipes with an alternative without researching a recipe first; I don't want to be responsible for your cake-turned–step stools!) It's almost like you're cheating when you use it. I think I am getting away with sugar robbery, and one day I will get caught. Shh, don't tell the sugar cops, but go out and get some.

"I happen to know everything there is to know about maple syrup! I love maple syrup. I love maple syrup on pancakes. I love it on pizza. And I take maple syrup and put a little bit in my hair when I've had a rough week. What do you think holds it up, slick?"

Okay, I had to throw that one in there (Jeremy Grey in *Wedding Crashers*) because I adore maple syrup. It has a strong flavor, which means you can't use it in everything, but it makes a great substitute for white sugar when possible. It's awesome on pancakes, of course, and it has great health benefits. Make sure you purchase 100 percent maple syrup, not just something that is flavored with maple.

Date sugar, turbinado sugar, and brown rice sugar are just a few more examples of alternatives to white sugar. Why do white sugar and high fructose get such a bad rap? Because they deserve it, of course! They are products that go through a big refining process, and they offer no nutritional value. This means they give us those empty calories. (Without going into great detail, just trust me on this one. If you don't, research it.) We are eating and drinking more sugar than we ever have in this country. Are we surprised that we have more health problems than ever before also?

Sugar isn't the only problem for our bad health, but it is a big one. Make sure it isn't a problem in your house, and try asking your sweetie to share you also; it worked for me.

— 24 —

"You can't show up at someone's house with Ring Dings and Pepsi!"

– 24 –

"You can't show up at someone's house with Ring Dings and Pepsi!"

Who doesn't love a good dinner party? I know we love to entertain in our home. Having friends and family over is one of my joys in life. We recently invited family over for a fried chicken and waffle brunch. It was our cheat day, so we could "afford" to have the fried chicken, and the whole-wheat waffles were served with toppings like fresh and cooked fruits. Blueberry compote, apple preserves, strawberry ricotta, thyme and raspberry syrup, macerated blackberries, and whipped cream were some of the side dishes I prepared. The cool thing about them is that I made many of them days before the party to lighten the load. All that had to be done the day of was fry chicken and heat maple syrup; my guest made their own waffles to order.

As easy as it was for me, it still was a fair share of work. We had nineteen guests in all. You could serve nineteen bowls of cereal and feel a bit overwhelmed.

Which brings me to the point of this Thing: have a party, and have your guests do all of the work. Not the dishes, but the cooking. Plain and simple, have a potluck. It is an easy way to have a nice party with friends and is less stressful than doing it alone.

And have your kids help out. Make this fun and educational. Leave the entire menu up to the kids so they can begin to entertain at a young age. Adults like to entertain, and children will, too, especially if there are young people there they can relate to. Kids like to feel like adults sometimes, so give your children a set of parameters to stay within and watch how creative they can be. Of course, the meal has to be healthy. Maybe you can give them a certain ingredient that has to be used in their dish, and they have to come up with the rest. Or you could exclude the use of other ingredients. It will be a challenge that the entire family can be involved in. Remember, it should be fun.

Have the kids help create a theme, and have everyone follow that theme. Italian, American Southern, childhood favorites, spicy food, pizza, tacos, or a sandwich or Panini party—these are just a few examples of types of parties you and your kids can host. Of course, you want to let everyone know what you are doing so you don't repeat dishes, but the key is to have fun and ensure variety.

The children should be able to invite other children from school, a cool way to get know your child's friends and their parents. If it is a success, you can start a trend. Hopefully, the next party will be at another's house. Of course, hosting your own party can be an easy invite for a family to accept, a bit more comfortable than you asking the parents of your kid's friend to host if you've just met them. Even if you just allow your children to pretend to host a dinner party in the house with you being the guest, that will be a lot of fun also!

You and your kids can also require that guests bring a dish that has no more than a certain amount of calories or fat per serving. Of course, this can be a little work, so reserve that one for a crowd that will be into it and will find it fun. The last thing you and your kids want to do is give guests a task they don't want and don't expect. You want people excited and eager when thinking about attending this event. If not, some may just show up with Ring Dings and Pepsi.

— 25 —

"I don't like potatoes but I love Tater Tots!"

– 25 –
"I don't like potatoes but I love Tater Tots!"

One Saturday morning in the Harper household, Daddy felt like making a big breakfast. Blueberry waffles and strawberry pancakes from scratch, homemade sausage, French toast from a homemade apple bread, warm homemade applesauce, fresh fruit parfait with granola, oven-roasted potatoes with fresh herbs, and freshly squeezed (by someone at the store) orange juice were all on the menu.

That wasn't the entire spread, either! Hey, I'm a chef, and when I get excited and inspired, I can get carried away; what can I say? I love preparing food, but what is even more exciting to me is when others enjoy what I have cooked. Making people happy through food is such a joy to me. It's why I love what I do; it's why I started cooking. Even though I didn't quite understand it at a young age, I was destined to entertain through food.

I'm sure you also like it when people actually enjoy what you prepare. How many times have you slaved over a meal, and the pickiest eaters of all, your offspring, immediately reject it with a look or even a taste. "Eww! What's that?" Sound familiar? It happens in my house, and I cook for a living! So it's worse for me sometimes. They mean no harm, but it can at times be hurtful to us. Do we cry and express to our children that they have just bruised our feelings? Not usually; we fire right back and tell them to eat it because this is what is being served! As you know, I encourage that, just without anger and with love. It's all a part of the process, we just have to learn about our children and understand how they eat.

As I write this book, my children are improving so much I can't tell you how happy I am. I thought for a while it would take years, but in just a few weeks, they have come a long way.

Rewind back to that big breakfast I made a few Saturdays ago. I was in the kitchen for quite some time, and I couldn't wait for them to see what I had done. I knew they would be ecstatic—or so I thought. For the most part, the food was well received. When I presented them with the potatoes, that's when the funny faces and negative comments ensued. Sarcastically, I asked Elijah what he would rather have than these wonderfully prepared potatoes, and he replied, "I don't like potatoes but I love Tater Tots!" I had to laugh. Even though I thought it was crazy that he would say that, I understood where he was coming from.

Yes, Tater Tots are made from potatoes, but to a kid, they are quite different. Let's start with the name. Tater Tots versus potatoes. That's easy; Tater Tots wins hands-down. No need to even discuss it. (I even like typing "Tater Tot," as you can see. It makes me feel warm, fuzzy, and childlike.) It's such a good name that Ore-Ida has a trademark on the word!

Look at it. It's all small and cute. Doesn't it make you smile? Okay, maybe I'm a little immature, but that's what I'm trying to tell you. I have a special connection with kids because of my inability to act like an adult, so my wife says. Seriously though, small foods are attractive to children. Our children are small and cute, so what would make us think that they want big, ugly foods?

We should take note from the big food companies that our children are so attracted to. These companies make billions of dollars off of us because they are smart and have smart marketing people. The only problem is they fill most of the food with too much fat, too much salt, and deadly preservatives. Use the marketing in your home to get your family to eat healthy. Who says you can't make little potato rounds in your house? I'm here to tell you that you can.

Make your healthy foods small and cute, and your children will eat them up! Also try to serve them in small portions, and the task of eating will be less daunting. Make a design on the plate and let your kids have fun with their fun. Try sticking fruit and vegetables on skewers. For some reason, there is something about eating food on a stick that intrigues us all, including kids. Cut foods in ribbons using a peeler; zucchini and squash are great for this. I'm guessing that your children loves french fries, so why not use their love of the fry shape to help with healthy eating? Get yourself a crinkle-edged knife and use it on carrots or parsnips. The list goes on and on.

Take away the garbage that is in a ton of little foods you find at the grocery store, and you may be left with some clever ideas about how to make healthy food cute for your children.

— 26 —

"Return to the root and
you will find the meaning."

— 26 —
"Return to the root and you will find the meaning."

I vaguely remember when I first showed my children a whole raw chicken. I was in the kitchen cutting it up, and they hit me with the proverbial "Eww! What's that?" I was shocked and disappointed at the same time. Shocked because even though they were fairly young, I thought they were old enough to know what a frickin' chicken was! They ate so many chicken nuggets; I thought they would have surely known what a chicken looked like. I mean, I am a chef, and I do cook raw food all the time. How can my kids be so repulsed by wholesome food?

The disappointment wasn't directed towards them; I put it back on myself. After all, they were three or four years old, and everything they had in their tiny little worlds consisted of what my wife and I had exposed them to. So if they didn't know what a chicken looked like, it was because I hadn't shown them what it was. I was the one with the tools and the knowledge to be able to introduce good food to the family.

As you have probably heard through the grapevine, restaurants can be pretty demanding. Between my two-hour commute to work and the hours spent at the restaurant, I was never really home for a good portion of my kids' lives. We make our choices, and I'm not here to question anyone's commitment to family or work. What I will say is that with those choices come sacrifices, and we have to be aware of the consequences. I made a choice to work like a dog and be away from home for days on end. I chose to sleep in my office sometimes because I was too tired to drive home and had to be right back in a few hours anyway.

I have had what some may call success in my professional life, and I am forever grateful for my experiences and what they have taught me. I am also aware of the consequences of my actions. While I was away, my children would ask for me like I worked in another country. When I got home, they would be asleep. When I left for work in the morning, they were asleep. When I did get a day off or had to just work the night, I didn't make time for my family because I was tired, and they let me rest. My wife would take my children out for the day and they would maybe go to the mall or out on the town. What would they eat? Junk, for the most part. I wasn't home when they came home from school to ask about food choices. I wasn't home to help pack school lunches and lend my expertise. I was never home to help cook dinner. I rarely went grocery shopping, so I didn't have any input in the products we had in the house. I tried to change the ways of the house, but I couldn't because I wasn't really "there."

I tell you this story only because it is my experience with living a hectic life. I know you live a pretty busy life—most of us do. But there comes a time when you have to make a choice and sacrifice something. Why do we choose to sacrifice the health of our families so often? I don't know, because I did the same thing. But I have made a change. I think you want to make a change, too, which is evident by you reading this far in the book. (By the way, thank you very much.)

The choice I have made is to teach my family what I know about food and how amazing it is. This starts with teaching them what real food actually is. We all know that children are explorers and investigators; we should use that to help them make healthy choices for life. After my kids "ewwed" the chicken, I made them come over and inspect and work with the bird. Of course, they were a little grossed out at first, but eventually they found it kind of cool.

I have written another Thing that encourages you to get your children in the kitchen and cook with you, but I want to take it a step further with this one. Great cooks respect their food, plain and simple. I feel like the more you know about your food, the more you will appreciate it, especially if that food gave its dear life for us to enjoy a meal. I take my cooks to farms and fisheries to actually see the work that goes into getting product through the back door. I encourage you to try that tactic with your family. I know you have a busy life, but it would be great if you could make the time.

Riding through this beautiful country, we have often stopped on the highway to look at the cattle that graze the farms. Because of the smell, we can't stay for long, but we just talk for a little bit about how those beautiful animals will soon be our dinner. Please spare me the "that's-so-cruel" talk—that is reality, and we should let our children in on the truth. It's not like I am taking them to the slaughterhouses! I like for them to see how hard the farmers work to provide for their families. Just a quick reminder every now and then about where your child's food comes from can go a long way, and it can also teach them how they should enjoy it from the source without so many additives and preservatives.

Fishing, crabbing, and even hunting are great methods for your children to connect with nature and their food. The easiest introduction to the source of their foods is to visit a fruit and vegetable farm. Have you ever picked and eaten a fresh strawberry in July? Have your children? If not, you are missing one of life's pleasures. Picking fresh fruit and vegetables can be so fun and very educational. It surely teaches us about where our food comes from, and I think that eases our children's minds when it comes to trying new foods. There are plenty of Web sites that can direct you to the farms in your area that will allow you to pick your own food. Some farms even have restaurants where you can buy the fresh food prepared on a plate.

At minimum, try to visit a farmers' market first. Farmers' markets are fun, and the farmers bring the food to your neighborhood. Encourage the children to ask questions. I find that the farmers are generally very open to discussing their products. Give your children spending money at the farm or the market, and watch them have fun picking out fresh, healthy food.

If that doesn't work for you and your family, try youtube.com or just Google "farming," and I'm sure you will get some great pictures and videos. Even though that may not be the best way for some to understand, it may be a great start for others. The key is to start teaching our youth about where their food comes from, no matter the means. It all starts with a choice. Commit the time and effort you feel is necessary, and make it happen.

Finally, I also suggest you teach your kids about where the junk comes from. Do a little research on some of the unrecognizable terms that you read on labels, and see what your family thinks about that!

— 27 —
Let them cook!

— 27 —
Let them cook!

L et's face it, our biggest challenge lies in getting the kids to open their minds to eating healthy foods. Whether it is vegetables, meats that aren't fried, or fresh fruit, trying not to get our kids to immediately reject it is tough and often very frustrating. I face the same challenges in my home that you do. But what has helped us over the years is allowing the children to have a hand at cooking. Whether you are starting with young ones or teens, there is something fun to do in the kitchen that can help with the family's eating habits.

We as a people tend to reject new things in our lives, especially food. We generally aren't adventurous enough when it comes to change and variety on a daily basis, and I think the reluctance comes from our experiences as children. This is why I suggest we "return to the root" of foods and allow our kids to visit farms, grow their own foods, cook in the kitchen, and, at minimum, help us shop. These experiences will be building blocks for that valuable moment when for the first time you see them apply the skills that you have been teaching them. Even more important, your children will be equipped with tons of smarts to help them with future choices.

Just the other day I made scones with Leah, and we had a great time. (It gets testy in the kitchen sometimes, but it was still fun and educational.) I believe we saw a scone in a store a few days prior, and she asked for one. I asked her if she would like to make her own, and she was all in for that, of course. We started by going to the store to gather the ingredients that were in the recipe. As we shopped, I helped her make changes to the recipe so we could make it healthier. All-purpose flour was in the recipe, and we substituted organic whole-wheat pastry flour. As opposed to heavy cream, we decided to use

2% milk. White sugar was replaced with turbinado sugar, and we added some ground flaxseed to finish it off.

That shopping experience was definitely helpful for our eating lifestyle, but it was worth even more for our relationship. My kids aren't model citizens at the grocery store all the time, but times like those make me happy to be a parent. I wish you the same.

On to the healthy cooking!

In the kitchen there are always limits to what your kids can do. I like to teach my children how to properly use a knife when they're as young as four or five years old. (Tamara goes bonkers when she finds out, but that's why someone invented earplugs, right?) Of course, I help them and hold their hands (so you chill out, too, and put the phone down and tell the child protective services that you have the wrong number). We started out using a butter knife to cut strawberries; it can even be a plastic one. Tasks like stirring foods in bowls, measuring ingredients, cracking eggs, and gathering the food out of the refrigerator or cabinets are all great for children.

As the children get to work with the product, we ask them questions to see whether they remember why the food is healthy for us.

"Why do we use whole-wheat flour, Leah?" I might ask while she mixes the dry ingredients together. A little unsure, she might respond, "Because it has fiber?" She may get it right, or maybe not, but if she hears it enough, it will begin to stick and make sense in her daily life. I strongly believe that the more you can actually put a name and a face with something, the less likely your kids will be to reject it, especially if they understand where it comes from and how to handle it. We talk about kosher salt versus iodized salt, white sugar versus turbinado sugar, fresh fruit versus canned, and so on. Of course, Leah and I weren't having this long, drawn-out conversation during cooking because that would make it boring and she would never come back. These are talks we have over time, and I might bring up a couple when we cook together. You can judge your child's interest, though, and if they are interested, keep going. But if your child begins to get frustrated and isn't really into the talking, you should probably back off. The key is to have their hands in food and for this to be a fun time.

The scones turned out great, but I have to be honest with you, she wasn't entirely thrilled with them. She did try them as did the entire family. She said they were good but she just didn't want a lot, which was okay with me—it was a great lesson. She had a great time rolling out the dough, cutting the scones, and then brushing them with milk. At the table she couldn't wait to explain to Elijah and Tamara what she had made. Add all of that on top of the knowledge she gained, and it was a success. Remember, we want our children familiar with many types of foods so they can be smarter than before. I think that goal was accomplished with Leah.

I am a chef, as you know, and many of my friends think that my profession gives me an edge in the kitchen with my kids. I would have to disagree in a big way. My cooking skills and knowledge of food are no match for the skills of a seven-year-old and a ten-year-old. Teaching people is another skill that has nothing to do with food. I wish I was a better teacher and am learning how to be, but it is definitely a challenge.

One of the keys to teaching well is to find your student's motivation and use it to help them learn. That's easier said than done, especially when you're a teacher to someone else's kids, and there are hundreds of them! Luckily, we only have the children in our home to worry about. Be patient in the kitchen with your children. I have to remind myself of the same thing. If I am in a rush and know that I don't have the patience, I will tell them that I will cook alone to avoid any testy moments.

(May I take this moment to apologize to all of my teachers that I caused heartache to. I feel your pain now.)

Remember to exercise your child's inner "Chef Rock" and let 'em loose!

~ 28 ~
"Constant dripping
hollows out a stone."

– 28 –

"Constant dripping hollows out a stone."

Don't use the "d" word; utilize one-pot cookery; take the kids shopping; go visit a farm; stop eating at fast-food places; get out and move a bit; and a bunch of other Things are what I am suggesting that you do to get your family on the healthy track. If you realize that you can use all 44 Things in your life, the thought of implementing them may be a bit overwhelming at first. Soon after you begin reading this book, my words may begin to be reminiscent of Charlie Brown's teacher's voice.

How many "d" words have you tried that ended up failing because it was too much to keep up with? It isn't just with eating—many times when we try to change things in our lives, we get in over our heads, and after a little while, we give up and go back to our old ways. I know I have done it tons of times in my life. I would hate for that to be the case with this book, so I offer you the following advice: take it easy.

I love the title of this Thing because it is such a study in patience and persistence. We live in such a fast-paced world, and too often we need "it" now. You have a beautiful life ahead of you; there is no need to rush. Every goal must start with one step. You should be proud of every step you take; congratulate yourself, and move on to the next goal. Maybe you will plan to change your food life on a weekly, monthly, or even quarterly basis. Whatever the goal, just make sure you have one, and remember that there is no quick fix. Healthy eating is not just about the food—there are so many other factors involved, and change takes time. If you can handle a heavy load, I surely think you should load yourself up with more change, but only if you can accept it in your life. Unhealthy eating is the stone, and your new habits are the drip. Keep going, and before you know it you will have punched right through that rock!

So how can you track your progress? How about keeping tabs on what you eat? Write down everything you and your kids eat for a week and put it away somewhere. Vow not to look at it for a year. Yes, a whole year. After making a year of small changes, I guarantee you will be so proud of your family when you realize how far you all have come. Of course there will be setbacks and challenges, but that is all a part of the journey.

Use a tablecloth to track your accomplishments. Purchase a tablecloth that can be written on with some fabric markers or just use a disposable paper one. Every time your kids try something new or have an eating breakthrough, write it on the cloth. When you run out of space, just start another! After a few months, it will be fun to go back and look at all of the different foods you all have enjoyed as a family.

Don't despair that you can't immediately make everything better. You can always make one thing better. –Ralph Marston

Vow to change one thing about your cooking or eating per day, week, or month. I would love to be able to say that you can implement all of the tools in this book immediately, but it just isn't likely. Not because you aren't capable—it's just that that's not how we as people operate. Change takes time, and we must remember that when trying these Things out on our kids. Start with one Thing, and when it is a part of your lifestyle, move on to the next one.

— 29 —

This doesn't taste good, but it's healthy for me?

~ 29 ~

This doesn't taste good, but it's healthy for me?

I never understood how rice cakes made it on the market. They stink. I have never tasted a rice cake that I liked. All of you health nuts who swear by rice cakes, save your e-mails trying to convince me of the brands that are awesome. I ain't buying it, literally and figuratively.

It is amazing to me when I hear about foods that are supposed to be good for us but lack taste. How can we be expected to eat healthy when many of the foods that are suggested taste horrible? I say we can't.

You can probably deduce that I am a chef who likes full flavor in his food, as both a consumer and a cook. I can't even imagine telling any of my guests, "This doesn't taste all that good, but it sure will help your health!" You should eat foods that get you excited about wanting to eat them! Your children should get excited about what they are going to eat. Don't they already? My children get so excited about their meals—not all of them, but we feed with flavor all of the time. When your children know you are ordering pizza, how many cheers do you get? You feel like a superhero who has just saved the city from doom. Bottom line: cook and eat food with flavor, and you have won half the battle.

Before you think I just endorsed eating junk food, slow your roll and keep reading. The trouble with many of us is that we haven't learned or been taught what food tastes like and how we can make it more flavorful. Sure, many people think cauliflower is not tasty, but that's probably because we have trained ourselves to think that way. I was recently listening to a culinary student go on and on about how she despised the smell of artichokes and therefore wouldn't eat anything with artichokes in it. One day, she was eating a dip that she thoroughly enjoyed and couldn't help but notice that her friends were having a good laugh while she devoured it. As you can probably guess, they knew it had artichokes in it. When they told her, she said something like, "I knew it had something in there that I didn't like." After that, she didn't eat another bite because the thought of eating artichokes disgusted her. All of this dates back to when she smelled a can of them for the first time and couldn't stand it. Who knows, they could have been spoiled, but she was forever turned off by that one experience.

We have to train our children and ourselves to recognize and appreciate flavors, textures, and aromas. Once our kids can recognize the great qualities of food, they will begin to appreciate them and understand their importance. That may sound like a bunch of foodie talk, but it is actually quite simple. Having the conversation about the food while you prepare and eat it is all that it entails. Recognizing the sweet and sort of milky and nutty flavor of cauliflower is a good beginning when dealing with the vegetable. Encourage your children to taste fruits and vegetables raw, then compare them to the cooked flavor after they have been prepared. Roasted cauliflower with a bit of olive oil and a touch of salt can be much tastier than raw cauliflower. I do think some raw foods are tasty and great for you, but there is a bunch of magic that happens when you apply seasoning and heat.

If you are a junk-food junkie and your kids are too, that's okay, because you are here to change. I don't want you or your family to eat food that doesn't taste good, but you have to meet me in the middle and try to understand what good-tasting food really is. Cook with fresh vegetables, healthy oils, fresh herbs, awesome spice, and the right amount of sea or kosher salt, and you will begin to recognize and appreciate great tasting foods that are excellent for your body.

You love pizza, and so do I. Make your own dough and use whole-wheat flour to add the healthy punch you need. Low-fat cheese, fresh tomatoes, fresh herbs, and leaner meats can help turn one of our unhealthiest joys into a healthy indulgence. Do you use ground beef in your tacos or pasta dishes? We do, and we love it. Most people would write on to tell you that ground turkey is an awesome substitute, but turkey sure ain't ground beef, no matter how you cook it. So if you love ground beef, use a leaner grade. Most of us normally purchase the beef labeled 80/20, meaning it is 80 percent meat and 20 percent fat. That's a lot of *gordo,* my friends, even if we do drain it off after browning. Purchase 90/10 or even 95/5, and that will help you with your fatty, beefy dilemma. Sure, the leaner meats costs more money, but you get more meat, and isn't that what we want? Also, if it helps your health, why would you care that it costs a dollar or so more a pound? If a few bucks in the grocery store bothers you, compare it with the hospital bills after having a stroke.

Life is too short to kill your food by not enjoying flavor, and life's also too valuable to devour food that kills you. Eat well and be happy, my friends.

— 30 —
"Let there be work, bread, water, and salt for all."

– 30 –
"Let there be work, bread, water, and salt for all."

I would like to dedicate this Thing to the honorable mayor of one of the greatest cities in the world. Mayor Michael Bloomberg of New York City, this one's for you.

Recently, the people running New York City have been determined to take on some of our biggest foes. They banned cigarettes indoors, and then out went the deathly trans fats. After having success with those two campaigns, the bigwigs in NYC got a little "chesty" and decided to take on their biggest enemy yet: salt. In short, they believe that if we reduce our salt intake, fewer of us will die of heart disease, and health care costs will be reduced. Mayor Bloomberg is leading the National Salt Reduction Initiative (NSRI) that proposes reducing salt in foods sold in the city and other places across the country.

State assemblyman Felix Ortiz took the initiative a step further and proposed that no restaurant in the state use salt at all! Under this bill, if the chef reaches for the kosher salt in your restaurant, he will be slapped with a $1,000 fine. Does he know that NYC is *the* restaurant capitol of the world, and that omitting salt from recipes would make dishes flavorless?

I will say that after reading the NSRI plan a bit more in depth, I recognized that it has great intentions and seems to target packaged foods in a big way. I think that is awesome because we need someone to stand up and reject the garbage that is being sold to us and our children in packages. But much of the media coverage has been about the use of salt in restaurants. I wouldn't have written this book if I didn't think there is a huge need in this country to curb deaths from heart disease. Salt is not the enemy, though—as a matter of fact, salt is our friend. We just have to know how to use it.

I often find myself speaking about salt to my

audience because, as simple as it is, salt remains a mystery to many of us. I won't give you a boring foodie-like take on salt; I just want to give you some pointers on how to use salt in your kitchen as it pertains to cooking healthy for your children.

The purpose of salt is to enhance flavors. Salt also regulates yeast in baking products, but in general, we should use it to bring out the goodness of everything we eat. There is not one thing I can think of that I do not use salt in. Without salt, food is bland, unexciting, and flat.

I encourage you to use salt, but not as a "flavoring," so to speak. When I was young, we used to have a bottle of McCormick's Season-All in the cabinet at all times. What did we use it on? Everything. It is named Season-*All,* right? (I should say it *was* named that because McCormick's has discontinued it.) Similar products contain a high amount of salt, and that taste is what we have come to think of as food being flavorful. If you taste the salt when you eat food, then it has probably been oversalted. I know that may break some of your hearts, but I have to tell you the truth.

We are such a busy people; we eat on the go on a regular basis, and we have to have everything conveniently prepared to fit our lifestyle. Take a look at how much sodium is in the foods we eat. That's where the health issues come from: processed and packaged foods. Even some of the "healthy" stuff is loaded with copius amounts of salt. Cut back on the processed foods, and you'll be cutting back on your salt intake.

I don't like to use iodized salt. I prefer kosher salt when I cook. "Kosher" refers to the way it is processed and contains no preservatives and therefore has a very clean taste. Kosher salt is easier to grab with your fingers because of the large crystals. This may sound a little weird, but it is less salty than regular salt, so you use less with the same or better effect.

Sea salt is a very broad term that usually means the product has come from evaporated seawater that has been unrefined. It also has a clean and fresh taste to it. Because it comes from the sea and isn't processed like other salts, it still has the natural minerals in it, which is why many people say it is the healthiest salt of them all.

There are tons of other salts that are far more expensive than these. I won't go into them here, but if you are interested, just search the Internet for different types of salt.

Don't be afraid of salt, be afraid of Felix Ortiz's proposed bill. Yes, obesity is a problem. Yes, heart disease is our biggest problem. But people who tell you that salt isn't okay to consume is our problem too. Eat whole and fresh foods, and season them well. Cut out the packaged and overprocessed garbage from your life, and you will immediately see and feel a change.

— 31 —

"I'm going to make him an offer
he can't refuse."

– 31 –
"I'm going to make him an offer he can't refuse."

There are certain things kids just don't understand and don't want to take the time to try to understand, either. In a short while, you will be done reading this book, and you'll be loaded with energy and knowledge to change your family's eating habits for a healthy future. Armed with new knowledge and enthusiasm, you will have nothing that can stop you—except for when your child refuses to eat, of course. You deal with that now, right? Plan to deal with it more, my friend. I have taken a look at a few of the "expert" books and references on this subject, and some of them paint this picture that all will be well in your land when making change.

One Web suggestion went something like this: Tired of feeding your children unhealthy and grease-laden French fries? We have the perfect alternative! Purchase a crinkle-cutter and cut some healthy carrots to look like fries, and your child will be delighted at the chance to eat a carrot fry!

Jinx, you owe me a drink, because we all said "yeah, right!" at the same time. Don't get me wrong—crinkle-cut carrots are an awesome, healthy, and cute treat, but they sure aren't a substitute for fries, baby. My point is that I understand the real challenges we face when it comes to making healthy change to your family's eating habits. I won't give you the impression that it will be totally easy. There will be times that you will want to give up, but don't give in; some of the tips I have to offer you can help.

As you have read already, I am a firm believer in sticking to your guns and not budging on the meal options. You cook what you cook, and I don't suggest you prepare an alternative for your child who doesn't want to eat. However, that can lead to some heavily spirited battles at the table that can be taxing on everyone involved. I love for my family to eat at the table together, and we also prefer to leave the table together. Well, that doesn't work if Elijah or Leah stage a boycott of the day's nourishment. Neither Tamara nor I will sit at the table for hours on end forcing them to eat. As stern as we may be, a little treat goes a long way—my kids don't eat vegetables and new foods faster than when a sweet is offered after dinner.

Keeping with the healthy life change, you can't offer a Krispy Kreme doughnut or a similar treat after they've eaten spinach. Offering something completely unhealthy after eating food that is good for you may send the wrong message. I've written an entire Thing on eating those sinful indulgences from time to time, so don't think there won't be room for the occasional "greedy" moment, but not as a treat on a regular basis.

Actually, doughnuts are a good example. They can be made healthy by simply not frying them. Of course, you can find tons of recipes for wholesome alternatives out there, and you can give them a try.

Fresh fruit with whipped cream and vanilla is another good dessert. Yes, I did say whipped cream, and yes, I do mean heavy cream. Remember, fat is not the enemy—too much of the wrong fats are our enemy. So if you plan to offer a rich dessert that has wholesome and healthy ingredients, you can make dinner a little lighter. The incentives are endless.

We tend to think of food when offering treats, but that's not all we can use to motivate our children. My son, Elijah, loves to log on to the Net to catch up on cartoons that he can't watch on television. We offer him thirty minutes on the Net if he eats all of the food in time. But we always try to tie his accomplishment to something educational. If he gets on the Net after eating broccoli, he may have to do a quick Internet search on broccoli and report what he found out. This way, we tie in the importance of eating great foods to his access to entertainment. Whatever your child loves, use it to get him through eating food on occasion. Be careful not to overdo it, though. You will set a precedent that your child will expect something for doing what he should be doing anyway.

Just think about your daily life and how often you treat yourself for doing something that is your responsibility. Did you work hard this week for your family, and you feel owed a manicure or end-of-the-week cocktail? Well, you are supposed to work for your family, but doesn't it feel great to have a reward to remind you of your accomplishments? I bet it would feel even better if someone else got you a reward for your accomplishments. Your kids feel the same way.

By the way, if you don't get a chance to be congratulated, I would like for you to put this book down and close your eyes for a moment. Think of all of your accomplishments, and hug yourself as hard as you can. I appreciate you and I believe that you are amazing. I hope you know that you are.

— 33 —

Hire a personal chef!

~ 33 ~
Hire a personal chef!

And by that, I mean that you add another hat to your collection and become your family's personal chef. By all means, if you can afford a personal chef, go for it. Personal chefs who don't live in are not as expensive as you may think, and I encourage you to support your local chefs every chance you can.

I have done a little personal chef work, and it is actually a great job. Most people who need personal chefs are really busy individuals or families who love to eat great food but feel they don't have the time to cook, or they just don't want to cook. Sounds like anyone you know? Yeah, sounds like almost everyone these days. Personal chefs have an extensive consultation with their client and then compose a menu for them to order from, or they already have a menu from which their clients choose meals. After the selections are chosen, the chef will prepare the food and package it to be frozen or refrigerated. When the client is ready to eat, they heat up the meals and enjoy.

When you are cooking healthy for your children every night, it can become a bit much if you don't act like a personal chef. The process starts when the food comes home from the grocery store. Carve out a day in which you have a few extra hours to set your family up for healthy eating success.

If you plan to have spaghetti on Monday, go ahead and cook the meat sauce, cool it down, and then refrigerate it so it is ready to go. Is chicken on your radar one day this week? Try cooking your chicken and cooling it down to be enjoyed later. Sure, fresh is usually better, but the point is to have wholesome foods, even if they are prepared another day. What will usually happen when you are short on time and driving home after sitting in traffic? You probably reach for the takeout coupons or make some quick meal that isn't as good as it could be. This is especially the case if the kids are home alone or if your partner doesn't even know where the kitchen is. How great would it be to tell them to just heat up the meal you have prepared already? By the time you get home, they will have a plate waiting for you! Even though you have cooked it, it will feel like someone else cooked for you. Having healthy foods around helps us avoid making rushed decisions when we are hungry.

You don't have to make whole meals, either; breaking food down for future use also helps. If you will be eating a lot of ground beef or turkey during that week, go ahead and brown it with oil, salt, and pepper before you put it in the fridge. Cut up onions, garlic, peppers, carrots, or any vegetables and fruits that don't brown to make them easier to eat and use later on. Just think of what you use often and try to think ahead to how it would be easier to cook if you had some of it prepared already.

If all else fails, just hire me.

– 33 –
Just don't get caught.

– 33 –
Just don't get caught.

Many times in a restaurant environment, the employees tend to eat whenever we can and whatever we can. It isn't uncommon to see a cook standing over a bowl of what appears to be mashed potatoes and chicken with gravy a few minutes before service starts. You would think that the cook is guarding the grub with his or her life after watching them suck the meal down in two minutes.

Jacques F. is a phenomenal chef, a great mentor, and an awesome human being. I worked under Jacques for quite some time, but as my career grew, he would always find a way to lend me pieces of priceless information. I remember working in Washington, D.C., and not feeling too inspired under my current chef. I told Jacques my feelings, and he urged me to stay. In the meantime, he invited me to work with him in Culpeper, Virginia, on my days off. Even though our restaurants were about ninety miles apart, I jumped at the chance.

One day at his place I witnessed something that changed my outlook on many levels. There was an older dishwasher working lunch, and Jacques caught him eating leftovers from a guest's plate. Jacques instantly went off! Now, listen, I have seen him make grown men cry over the years, but this was a different kind of scolding. He pulled the guy aside and instructed him to never do that again. Aside from the health concerns of eating after other people, the chef was more upset that the dishwasher felt like he couldn't have a fresh meal for himself, and that this would happen in his kitchen. From then on out, the dishwasher ate what he wanted, and he felt better about himself and his boss; it was evident in his work.

After experiencing that, I vowed I would always allow my cooks to enjoy food in the same manner the guests do. Of course, we can't sit down and have a seven-course meal laden with lobster, truffles, and veal every week, but when it's time to enjoy a meal, we do it well, and we treat ourselves with the same respect as we treat the guests. When I eat a burger, I want an awesome burger, and I want to sit and enjoy it.

When your family begins this new healthy eating and living Thing, one of the best tactics is to remember who you are and what you like. The key to success is occasionally diverting from your lifestyle. When you divert, or should I say cheat, make sure you do it well and don't get caught.

I have given you several tips and tools that I think will help you get your cooking and eating on the healthy fast track. At the end of it all, the fact remains that we like what we like. There are several thousand burger chains in this country for a reason: we like burgers. We like fatty and sugary foods. Remember step one, acceptance: I know who I am and I don't run from it. The key, however, is not to run towards it every day. Choose how often you plan to cheat and stick to it. If you choose to take your family out on a cheat day every week, that's a great start. Just think, we generally eat twenty-one meals in a week, and if you splurge on two, that's ten percent or less that you eat garbage. Or you can look at it on the flip side: you eat healthy 90 percent of the time. That's pretty darn good.

Of course the "experts" tell us that eating healthy 100 percent of the time is best, but that thinking isn't realistic, nor is it fun. Would God have given birth to the culinary mastermind that is Paul Prudhomme and then bless him with the inspiration to stuff a turkey with a chicken? Would the Creator then give him the motivation to stuff a duck in that chicken that is stuffed in the turkey if He wanted us to always eat healthy? I say no, my friends.

Every Friday when we were younger, my mother would take us to a restaurant in Alexandria, Virginia, called the Ground Round, and we could get whatever we wanted. Lucky for us, kids paid the equivalent of their weight on some days, and on other days they paid their ages (in cents, with a zero tacked on the end). Otherwise, we wouldn't have been able to afford it. Even though my mother probably made us fast for three days to shed a few pounds before Friday, we were so excited about the experience.

I think if we know anything, it's how to cheat. But I'm sure you're asking what I mean when I tell you not to get caught. Getting caught is when you indulge in the "good stuff," but instead of eating foods prepared with love, you visit a deadly fast-food joint and call that cheating. That isn't cheating, that's getting caught. If you want a burger, visit a place like Five Guys that uses fresh, whole foods to make you happy. We grow up thinking a visit to the infamous burger place is a treat because of all the toys and the box that the meal came in. That's getting caught. Eating something that resembles a golden piece of chicken but is actually a ground-up "nugget" of chemicals and mystery is how you get caught cheating. If you want to eat fried chicken, eat fried chicken. Make your own and teach your children what great food should taste like. If you visit the grocery store to purchase a frozen apple pie and ice cream, you might be on the verge of getting caught. It's pretty easy and fun to make an apple pie, and your ingredients haven't been sitting in a freezer after traveling from the other side of the country. I'll also bet you'll find a local shop that makes whole-some ice cream, too, without all of the nonsense you read on many of the labels in the store.

I took the lesson from Jacques and ran with it. My cooks can eat whatever they want when I run a restaurant. Not like greedy idiots, but like culinary professionals who care about the food they consume. I would encourage you to embrace the fact that your children like certain foods. But teach them what good food should taste like, and help them from falling into the trap of loving fast-food that is riddled with trash.

What's beautiful about cheating is that it isn't something you do on a regular basis, so you are training yourself and your children that the food you are consuming today is just for today and that you have to get back on track tomorrow.

— 34 —
I never say never, but . . .

– 34 –

I never say never, but . . .

How many chefs have you heard tell you to never do something in order to achieve a perfect result? You can turn to a cooking show right now, and I will bet you that the program won't finish before some talking head will tell you to "never put cheese with fish" or "always use sea salt." I have learned the hard way to never say never. More times than not, when I utter the words "never" and "always," people rush to prove me wrong. And prove they do, because in a world of so many possibilities, there aren't many absolute truths.

Even though I am sure I will be flooded with e-mails attempting to prove me incorrect, I am pretty confident with breaking my own rule when I write this: if you want your children to eat healthy food, never cook anything in water and then serve it to them.

Of course, there are certain foods you can cook in water and then season or marinate them, but that's not what I mean. I do understand that there are certain meals that have steamed or blanched accompaniments to the entrée that create balance, but that's not what I mean, either. I am talking to all of you out there who have emptied a can of green beans into a pan and heated them, then served them to your kids. You should be arrested.

You often hear people say that they hate certain foods. In my profession, I hear it all the time. After asking why people detest certain foods, I find their distaste often comes from an experience that dates back to childhood. Do you really want to turn your child off to healthy food? You will if you don't begin adding flavor to food.

Don't misunderstand what I'm saying. Many people tend to think that flavor comes from some elaborate process that one attains only after years of

187

training. That's not it. Most whole and healthy foods have great flavor by themselves, they just need a little salt to bring them out. Salt and pepper go a long way. Use fresh pepper if you can; it tastes better than the product that sits on the shelf for months on end. Whatever you use, just use something.

— 35 —
Go raw

— 35 —
Go raw

I don't mean to act as if I am an authority on the raw-food movement, but I think that the health benefits are awesome and can help when you try to cook healthy for the kids. I am not a food scientist, nor am I trained as a nutritionist. I am a chef and I try to use common sense when I do things. Common sense says that if certain foods are great for us in their cooked form, then they have to be healthy in their raw form. Some say that cooked fruits and vegetables lose almost all of their nutrients, but I don't believe that for one second. I do believe, though, that the longer foods cook, the more the food loses some of its nutritional value.

Raw fruits and vegetables are extremely healthy for us and our children. The more we introduce raw ingredients to them, the more receptive our children will be to eating different types of foods. It's pretty easy to get our children to eat sautéed broccoli covered in cheddar cheese sauce, but how challenging is it to get them to consume that same broccoli fresh out of the produce section? Raw broccoli is one of the best vegetables on the planet. But I'm pretty confident in saying that most kids will choose a soft-cooked broccoli smothered in cheesy goodness every time. I don't think the key is getting your children to eat raw vegetables all the time—I believe that having a great balance between the two is the key.

Eating raw vegetables is also a great teaching tool for children to see and understand how food changes through cooking. Many times we grow up not knowing the process our food goes through before we actually eat it. Inviting your kids into the kitchen and encouraging them to taste raw food before you cook it can be an awesome way for them to appreciate the flavors and healthy benefits of food.

I also encourage my kids to taste as I cook the food so they can see and taste how it changes. They taste the oils, salts, peppers, and anything thing else that I cook with (except raw meat, of course). Do they like it all? Of course not. Are they budding food snobs? Hardly. All I want to do is get them comfortable with real, healthy, wholesome, and fresh foods. The more familiar they are with these foods, the more likely they are to try new foods.

Try to introduce a raw food every week or month to your kids; you might be surprised at how they will react. Don't feel the need to pair the foods with dip, either. (I mean really, what doesn't taste good dipped in blue cheese?) The goal is to broaden their palates by teaching them what the foods taste like raw; if you couple them with a fatty dip or sauce, it kind of defeats the purpose. Even if the dip is healthy, it still masks the taste. Of course, dips and sauces are awesome for raw food, but for the first time, try to feed them raw foods without condiments.

Raw foods tend not to fill you up as fast as

cooked foods, so be prepared to hear often "I'm still hungry" after your kids eat a ton of raw foods. This may be why more people haven't gravitated toward eating raw. I eat five or six times a day now, and eating totally raw may double that. That is a lot of work! This is why raw-food enthusiasts have a hard time trying to convince me to make the switch. But I do think that eating raw food is one of the best ways to live and can help our children live longer lives.

Recently, Tamara and I were candidates to be on Jerry Seinfeld's show *The Marriage Ref,* a funny show about using celebrities to help settle couples' disputes. We didn't make it on the show, but it was an awesome experience to even be considered, and we had fun. The casting for this show consisted of a crew coming to our home and filming our dispute that we needed Seinfeld and his friends to help re- solve. The lead casting producer was a woman who looked very youthful. After we spoke for a while, she revealed that she was fifty or so years old. We couldn't believe it. She really looked thirty-something. To make a long story short, her secret was eating raw foods. We had a good talk about it, and she sparked our interest. So I decided to experiment a bit.

When I eat raw fruits and vegetables, I feel great. When I feed my family a healthy breakfast with a bunch of raw goodies, we have awesome days. I have studied our behavior, and we do better when we eat more raw foods. On the flip side, when we eat badly, we feel bad. I even notice less gray hair when I have more raw food in my diet. It's pretty amazing. I have read plenty of stories of people overcoming major illnesses by eating raw, and I believe every bit of it.

I love eating animals too much to even think about converting to a total raw-food lifestyle. But I do know it can be the best thing for you and your children's health to at least occasionally try it.

— 36 —
Never hide food in food

– 36 –
Never hide food in food

You just read how I try to rarely use the words "never" and "always," and here I am using "never" again. Well, I'm breaking my own rule! (If you think that's crazy, wait until you read the next Thing!)

I don't care how much research is out there about hiding healthy foods in food you cook to get your children to eat healthier. That tactic stinks, if you ask me. I believe in allowing children to participate in their well-being. Someone once told me that the greatest gift you can give anyone is a sense of value, and I believe that stands true. Our children will feel amazingly valuable if they play an active role in their nutritional choices, especially when they begin to make great choices. In contrast, if you deceive children about what they are really consuming, it can be damaging and useless in the long run.

The suggestions of how to hide healthy food are endless, so I won't even begin to give them to you. Some people live by this practice and I can't knock it, but I am not going to do it, nor do I suggest you do it, either. What is the end result of years of hiding healthy food? I can't tell you specifically because I haven't done it, but I can guess that the children who receive it have no clue that they are eating healthy. So when you make cookies and blend in white bean puree to make them healthier, they think they are eating cookies like the ones sold in school or in the store. When faced with a choice on their own, those children will think that there is nothing wrong with eating cookies as a regular snack. "Mommy lets me eat cookies all the time, so it can't be bad for me."

If you puree carrots and use them as a way to hide nutrients in spaghetti sauce, do you think your child will just end up loving carrots? It's possible, but unlikely. What do we learn when kids say they hate a certain healthy food, but gobble it up when we hide it in other foods? I think we learn that the child has a mental block about the food and obviously will eat them when prepared properly. Many people would just continue to hide the food and be happy with that. What happens when they attend a sleepover or go away to summer camp? They will reject the food at first sight. Remember, our kids will eat most of their meals outside of the home for a great deal of their lives.

What's worse is that they could begin to distrust us. Tamara and I know our kids don't like some of what we say when it comes to setting rules, but we work on gaining and keeping their trust. I want my children to trust me, and I'm sure you do as well. I urge you not to deceive them to try to get them to eat healthy. Encourage your children to be adventurous and try new foods. Cook with flavor and love. Get excited about food, and eventually your children will follow suit.

~ 37 ~
Hide food in food

– 37 –
Hide food in food

Wait, wait, wait! Of course I know what I just said—I wrote it. Stick with me for a second, and I will explain why I break my own rules and contradict myself.

"Never say never" is such a good rule, because there is always at least one exception to the "never" rule. I still stand by what I just wrote in the previous Thing—don't hide healthy food in food and deceive your children about what they are eating. However, you *can* hide food in food; you just have to let them know about it.

I make foods with healthy ingredients all the time. Just the other day I had some carrots and pineapple that I didn't know what to do with. After doing a bit of research, I decided on muffins; everyone likes muffins, right? I made a carrot and pineapple muffin that I added agave nectar, flaxseed, and wheat flour to in order to make them healthier. They were awesome, and the kids killed them! Until I told them what was in them, that is. As soon as they knew there were carrots in them, they didn't want a second helping. It was disappointing because they had just devoured them a short while ago. It was a classic case of the mind taking over the taste buds. I was hoping they would see the lesson that they were psyching themselves out, but they weren't getting it. I made over a dozen muffins, and they weren't about to go in the trash, so I served them along with breakfast. They didn't like it, but they had to eat them. We also talked about the health benefits of the ingredients, and I think that may have helped, but they couldn't get past the idea that an actual muffin had carrots in it. *Carrots are those things that are served with chicken!* is what they were probably thinking. Just imagine if someone tried to serve you bacon-flavored ice cream—it wouldn't fit right in your mind.

(Well, I have had it, and it was pretty good. But the thinking is the same.)

This book has a lot of suggestions to get children involved in their food consumption, but I don't think it's feasible to have a lesson in gastronomy at every meal. You are embarking on a new lifestyle, so these are tips to help over many, many years to come. I just don't want you to think that I recommend you to ask for suggestions from your kids at every meal.

Go ahead and mix in mystery ingredients! You don't even have to tell them that you used something different. In many homes, healthy is the norm, and there is no need to explain healthy foods as different from the norm because they aren't. But I still think that talking about what you are eating is a great practice for any family.

If you do find the need to secretly put healthy foods in what you cook, just tell them about it after they eat it. Let their taste buds decide before their brains do.

– 38 –
Lights, camera, YouTube!

– 38 –
Lights, camera, YouTube!

Everyone wants to be a star, and that includes your child. We live in a world of Twitterers, MySpaceness, and Facebookies. I don't know about yours, but our children beg and beg to be involved in the social Internet revolution. A lot of parents, including us, keep them away from many of these outlets fearing that they could be exposed to danger and threats.

We recently shot a sizzle reel for our future reality show with Interface Media Group in Washington, D.C. (A sizzle or demo reel is kind of like a commercial that production companies use to sell the concept of a television show to networks.) The sizzle shoot was centered around my business and my family. I had a few meetings that were filmed, and then

I cooked with kids. There was a crew of about four people, and the kids couldn't have been more excited. It was a challenge to try to not get them to look into the cameras, but they did a phenomenal job in the end. When we watched the final cut at the studio, the kids watched it again and again. They were amazed to see themselves on TV cooking.

When we are at home and they play with the Webcam, they are just as amazed as they were when they saw themselves on *Hell's Kitchen.* To a kid, there is no difference, whether they are being filmed for real or not. Well, kids outside of Los Angeles, that is.

Use this excitement of being on a screen to your advantage. Use it as an outlet to educate and inspire your little ones. Let them host their own cooking show and post it on YouTube.com, if you're comfortable with that. Set some ground rules and modify the system as you progress. If they are going to have a cooking show, maybe it is all about healthy food and making treats that are good for you. Of course, it will be a little unorganized at first and maybe a bit unentertaining, but that is hardly the point. You want them to get really excited about the world of healthy food. Don't worry about them looking into the camera or making mistakes. When they get to watch the final cut, they will think they are the next Miley Cyrus or Keke Palmer, no matter what.

Cooking is sometimes a big deal, and I understand that may not work for you, so try something else. An episode can be as simple as fixing a bowl of cereal for breakfast. Your child can talk about the cereal for a few seconds and the health benefits of their choice. The milk can also be a great talking point. Remember, you just want them talking about healthy choices.

If you employ some of these tactics, how excited will they be to learn about new foods and how they can incorporate them into their show?

Even if they don't touch food at all while filming, many kids love to talk. Isn't that what the social networking boom is all about? People want a voice and want to stay connected. Use this climate to work for you and your family. Your child can just talk on camera about food and a healthy lifestyle. You could probably take a trip to the spa for a week if you allowed your child to sit in front of a camera for as long as they wanted!

When I was on *Hell's Kitchen,* I met a very interesting and amazing young man named Javier. Javier attended a high school where we had to cook for a hundred students and have them decide whose dish was the best. I cooked Kobe burgers, and Javier was the one student with the most questions. But he didn't ask questions as you might expect any other seventeen-year-old to; his questions seemed more to test me about my knowledge. He wasn't snobby at all; I could just tell the guy knew his food. I remember thinking, "Gordon has us cooking for a bunch of young food snobs; I'm never going to win!" (I did end up losing to Julia's grilled chicken and cheese sandwich with onion rings, so even if they were all foodies, it goes to show that good ole comfort food always wins.)

As it turns out, Javier was a budding food enthusiast. He is an awesome blogger, and you should check out his work at www.javiercabral.com; I'm sure you will enjoy it. I don't know the details of his childhood, but I do know the man loves food, and he had an outlet to express himself.

Just imagine what your kids can do with the proper tools and encouragement. I also want you to imagine what it can do for their enthusiasm when it comes to their eating habits. Tap into your children's excitement about media, and make it work!

— 39 —
Travel with a kitchen

– 39 –
Travel with a kitchen

One of the biggest challenges to our family maintaining a healthy lifestyle is when we hit the road. If you have traveled before, you know exactly what I mean. I'm not going to even get into how expensive it is while away on vacation or a weekend trip; that's another book entirely.

Just about every year since our children were three years old, we have traveled to one of the happiest places on earth, Disney World. Disney is an awesome vacation that we really look forward to every fall. The first time we visited, we stayed in some hotel about fifteen miles away from the parks that was pretty cool. It had all of the amenities and extras one would expect from a hotel in Orlando. We didn't realize until a couple of days in that our food options were seriously limited, though. There were some stores on the lobby level of the hotel that offered your regular run-of-the-mill quick convenience options along with a few different full-service restaurants. The kids' menus offered the ubiquitous chicken fingers, macaroni and cheese, and pizza. Of course, the vegetables offered were something like steamed broccoli. How exciting, right? We were hard pressed to get a healthy meal for our children that tasted good and was affordable. Because our other option was to order from the adult menu for the kids and have them split a regular entrée—which isn't always the healthiest route—we were probably spending anywhere from $70 to $100 a day on food and snacks that were far from healthy. So along with money, we were also low on energy.

We decided to be a little smarter the following year. We rented a hotel that had a kitchen in it and did all the cooking ourselves. Of course we set aside a little money for a few restaurant visits, because that's part of the vacation intrigue. But for the most part, we cooked all of our food ourselves. We started by going grocery shopping as soon as we checked into the hotel, because if we put it off, we would never have the energy to do it later. We didn't buy too much food because we didn't want to waste it or have to use a bag of oranges as our carry-on for the flight back. Even if we drove, we still limited the perishable items that we bought.

Vacation is supposed to be happy and memorable. The last thing you want is your kid not liking the food—especially pricey food—while on vacation. If your child likes a certain cereal and certain fruit, preparing it yourself helps you control that. I love breakfast restaurants just like anyone else, but they can't cook like me. Eggs are the one food that everyone thinks they have the perfect recipe for, and I'm no different. I'm probably not the best in reality, but I am for my family. Ever try to explain to your server how you or your family likes their eggs cooked? As the words come out of your mouth, you realize that no matter what you say, all of your eggs will be coming out however they cook them. When you have eggs in your kitchen, you control that. You also don't have to pay three bucks extra per person to use an egg substitute, either. The beauty is that you can keep things as normal as possible when it comes to healthy cooking, so your family can spend time having an awesome holiday.

You may lose some of the luster of what you get when stay at a "regular" hotel, but I believe it is well worth it. On vacation, we don't spend much time in the room anyway, so all we need is a nice bed to sleep in. Many of the hotels with kitchens are less expensive, so I believe it make sense for your wallet, also.

The reason it is so important to keep eating healthy on the road is because you can absolutely ruin much or all of the effort you have put in if you and your family go on vacation and grub on garbage for a week. Vacation is for having fun and trying different things, but that doesn't mean you have to be totally unhealthy. While we are away, we cheat probably every day, but we also load up on healthy food each day to balance it out. As a matter of fact, I think it is imperative that you cheat while away to help with healthy eating. It can send the message to your family that this cheating is not normal, and that you are doing this because you've earned it. If you visit a place like New Orleans and don't indulge in the local cuisine on a regular basis, let me tell you something: you ain't on vacation, my friend.

Even though some parks may frown on it, we take healthy treats to eat throughout the day. We may take a lunch break in the parking lot if we time it right. In the big parks, that isn't always practical, and no one wants to go all the way back to the car just to eat. The family wants to eat right now, not wait on cheap dad to dish out carrot sticks in the minivan. I get it. I suggest taking along something that travels well in mom's purse or in another bag. Nuts, dried fruits, healthy bars, and some vegetables are examples of what can help you stay on the healthy eating track while away.

Cooking on the road definitely helps with your goal of getting your family to eat right, but I've also found that it can help the getaway run a bit smoother. When you eat out or order room service, that can take hours away from the trip, especially with small kids. By cooking your own healthy meals, you can count on your family eating when you want and what you want. You have more time for each other and for actually having a retreat. All of your meals don't have to include multiple courses, either; they can all be one-pot dishes if that suits you best. We just want them to be healthy, substantial, and great-tasting, that's all.

Try it little by little and see how it goes. Try packing lunches on a weekend drive and see how you like it. If you're bold like me, you can just jump right in and start planning your next vacation now!

– 40 –

"Never doubt that a small group of thoughtful, committed citizens can change the world; indeed, it's the only thing that ever has."

– 40 –

"Never doubt that a small group of thoughtful, committed citizens can change the world; indeed, it's the only thing that ever has."

Many people don't believe they can change the world, and they don't realize that they already are doing so. Through action or inaction, the world is changed every day by what we do or what we don't do. I have been changing the world consciously for quite some time now. By typing these very words, the world will be altered. I know you also have the power to change the world.

As you can tell, I'm a pretty confident person, but I do have my moments of insecurity and feeling overwhelmed. In all of my confidence, I have learned a particularly valuable lesson, though: know when to ask for help, and actually ask for help. Like many men, I was raised to believe that asking for help was a sign of weakness, a sign that one had lost or was losing a battle. Men don't do that. The moment I put the kibosh on that thinking, life got a little better, to say the least.

Gladly, you are smarter than I am, because by reading this book, you have already acknowledged that you are unafraid to try new things or tap into the resources around you. When it comes to cooking healthy for your kids, I encourage you to go even further and make looking for new ideas a regular occurrence in your circle of friends.

Start a group that will change the world! Okay, maybe the world is a little ambitious, so in the meantime, start with changing your world. Tell your friends and family about your desire to cook healthy to bounce some ideas off of them. Meet on a regular basis. Start off small, unless you can handle an overwhelming amount of suggestions, feedback, and complaints. I have family and friends I wouldn't e-mail and ask to be a part of my group, either, just because I am fully aware of the negative vibe they would present to my mission. (If you are a friend or family member of mine and you just wondered whether I was writing about you, I probably was. I still love you, though!)

I always suggest starting off nice and slow; don't try to jump right in and overwhelm yourself. Invite two people or couples, and start from there. Too many people in your healthy cooking "summit" will force you to never do it again after experiencing the first bit of confusion. The same goes for the frequency and length of the meetings. Once a month or once every three months should suffice. If you want to do it less or more, go for it.

Okay, now what?

Once you have your crew assembled, you just share ideas and experiences about cooking healthy. *What worked for you? What new foods did you try since the last meeting? What tricks do you have? Any new recipes since we last talked? I can't understand why my child does (fill in problem that makes you pull your hair out); have you ever experienced this before?* I could think of at least twenty more questions that I've asked my friends and family. The goal is to just bounce ideas off of each other and see what comes back. We all need a fresh perspective—that's what change is about. Change, real change, requires you to open your mind to new things and have open conversations.

You may be surprised to find that you aren't the only one with the craziest eaters in the world. You will also be surprised at how many suggestions people have for you and also how you can help change another's life. It's all about having dialogue. Isn't that why Twitter, MySpace, and Facebook were all created—so we can stay connected and remain part of the "conversation"?

Speaking of the social networking sites, use those also. If you don't have anyone in your area, try connecting through the Internet to friends or family. Actually, I think it would be awesome to meet strangers and discuss solutions to your challenges of eating healthy. A fresh perspective is the most awesome thing ever. I live in Virginia, and the wonderful people of Oregon have products and techniques for eating healthy that I would have never thought of before speaking with them.

Your "summit" could be as easy as an e-mail with four questions on it that goes out when you begin. Hold discussions on Facebook, on Skype, or by snail mail, but by any means, just answer others' questions based on your experiences, and watch the change in your world.

─ 41 ─
Horror-movie food

– 41 –
Horror-movie food

Watching movies in the theater with the family is a classic pastime that we have come to love and cherish. Whether it's talking toys or witty donkeys, we flock to the big screen several times a year to take it all in. Even though you have to take out a loan against your 401(k) to actually see one movie a month, the films are well worth it. As I write this book, 3-D has totally taken over and is making its way into our homes. State-of-the-art theaters are phenomenal, and all of the costs of making and promoting a movie trickle down to us—and rightfully so. The end result is a movie experience that, for the most part, gets better every time we visit.

Based on the numbers, the genius of James Cameron has "touched" us with his films more than anyone else in the history of movie making. If you can't involve yourself in a James Cameron conversation, you are one of two things: stranded on an island for thirty years, or five years old. When you get rescued, chances are that *Avatar* will be the in-flight film on the way back home. Have you seen *Aliens?* Where did you see *Terminator?* How did you feel after watching *Titanic?* These are just a few questions that may arise when talking about the man and his work. I have another question, however, that you may not have pondered:

What were you eating?

Popcorn has to be what most of you are thinking. Popcorn is what I am thinking. We love those little warm, crisp-yet-airy kernels, especially when they're drizzled with salt and butter—although I'm pretty sure that the yellow, greasy liquid that smells like enchanting death is not butter. It smells good and the aroma makes us happy, but you have to admit that you are aware that soon after tasting a bit, it feels like your heart has slowed down a bit.

Or maybe your snacks of choice are hot dogs, nachos, chocolate-covered peanuts, colored candies, ice cream, or pizza that has been cooked in an oven in Cleveland and shipped to your local theater and reheated for your eating pleasure. Whatever it is, all of these offerings are crappy junk. A *medium*-sized popcorn with butter can have about 1,200 calories and 60 grams of saturated fat! Please read that last sentence again. I am not huge on counting calories as a mode to live by, but something about those numbers spells trouble. If I lay down fifty bucks for the tickets and then another thirty for food for my family, I don't want crappy food that is going to kill us. I hope you feel the same.

Instead of indulging in the offerings at the movie house, try eating at home before you go. Of course, there is nothing like reaching into the bag of salty and buttery goodness that's on Mom's lap while watching the newest flick, and I will get to that. What I'm talking about here is feeding your family before you go out to the cinema, because one of the worst ways to feed your little ones is at the movies.

My ten-year-old son can eat like me. Two hot dogs, popcorn, nachos, and a soda can cost us about $20. Even worse, it can cost him his life in the long run, and I just don't want to see that happen. We try to eat a meal before we go to prevent that from happening.

I can't condone taking money away from a business, in this case, the theaters, but I understand why people bring their own food sometimes. When you bring a product into a business that the business offers, you are preventing them from making a sale, and therefore you are taking money away from them. In restaurants, the same thing happens when people want to bring in desserts and wine. We charge you because if everyone did that, we would be out of business in a week. I do moan and complain about the costs of going to a movie, but I understand it, though. It costs a ton of scratch to run a theater. But if there are no healthy offerings and a family wants to bring some air-popped popcorn hidden in Mom's oversized BCBG bag, I can't blame them. I do feel like a movie just ain't a movie without munching on something, but I can't encourage my kids to eat crap every time they sit down to watch one.

Do we eat the food at the movies? Yes, sometimes. Remember, I am not a food snob. I don't encourage food snobbery. As a matter of fact, I think it should be a crime. But you can't offer your children this garbage regularly and expect them to eat your healthy food. Sure, we can cheat on occasion, but if you go to movies like we do and you eat there all the time, *Run, Fatboy, Run* won't just be a movie title—it will be the family mantra.

~ 42 ~

To whom it may concern: are you trying to kill our children?

– 42 –

To whom it may concern: are you trying to kill our children?

Cooking healthy for children is not just about tips, tricks, and recipes that you can employ in your kitchen. Healthy eating is a lifestyle, and there are so many elements in our environment that dictate how successful our children will be at sustaining a healthy lifestyle. I can't bring myself to write some blather about how you should try to cook like me and make everything healthy for your family. I have to be real with you and try to lend you some honest advice to help you win this battle. You aren't fighting your children, though—the struggle is with the many outside influences that affect your kids' decision making.

Millions of children eat two meals a day away from home when school is in session. Do you know what they are feeding your children? Do you automatically trust the school's kitchen to feed your child a proper, healthy meal? If you don't know, you should find out.

The schools are killing our kids, literally.

I am not an extremist using these words for shock value. Our children are unhealthier in this country than they have ever been before, and we as a people are dying younger because of our unhealthy lifestyles. As a matter of fact, the world is beginning to follow us. We live in the greatest nation in the world, in my opinion. We set many trends and standards, including our eating habits. These poor habits are beginning to spread to other corners of the world, and their citizens, too, are dying. Obesity is out of control, and I'm sure you know that because of your desire to seek out a little help.

One would think that the school systems we trust our kids to every day would feed them responsibly. Well, they don't. The Food and Drug Administration isn't our best friend, either. If they were, how could breakfast pizza fit into the recommended healthy food pyramid?

The only way to progress is to scream and shout from the mountaintops—in the form of a letter, of course. Write your school's principal, assistant principal, the superintendent, the mayor, the governor, your senator, your representatives, your president, and anyone else who you think needs to hear your message.

The message should be clear: stop hurting our children! Stop having garbage designed as healthy food fed to our children. Start committing more money, time, resources, education, and love to our children's food.

Have you eaten in your kid's cafeteria? I suggest you do so, and then write to them about your experience. However, some schools have awesome healthy options. You should write and congratulate those responsible for the good things with the same excitement and vigor that I encourage you to use when you shout about the garbage others are feeding your kids.

There is an old Yiddish saying, "To a worm in horseradish, the whole world is horseradish." I love that saying! Think of healthy eating as a horseradish. If your child is surrounded only by an abundance of healthy eating, that's all they'll know. We must do what we can to surround our kids with "horseradish" in and out of our homes.

— 43 —

Ban trans fats in your world

– 43 –

Ban trans fats in your world

Some years ago, before it was cast into New York law, we at B. Smith's Restaurant in D.C. stopped using trans fats. I was the chef at the time, and there was more and more research being done on trans fats that caught our attention. As much as I wish I could take total credit for it, I can't. It was a collective effort that took some thinking. B. Smith had three restaurants at the time, with one located in New York, New York, where there was a ban on trans fats looming. So we began to look more into what we were serving in all of the restaurants and how it affected our guests. As it turns out, these fats are pretty darn bad, and we were using a bunch of them.

In any event, we took trans fats off of the menu

and never looked back. I sat down with my sales representative from my main food vendor, and we worked out some great alternatives to our products that had trans fats in them. It raised our costs on many fronts. The products themselves cost more. Some of recipes changed completely because they relied on a product like margarine, which is laden with trans fats. We started using butter in those recipes, but you can't just substitute products in recipes and not expect change; they changed and not in a great way. We had to develop new recipes, new techniques, and a new thinking; it was one of those aha moments in my career. So why would the owners spend thousands of dollars on something that wasn't mandated in D.C.?

Because trans fats are deadly.

You should know by now that I don't think fat is the enemy. Most fat, at least. Trans fat is your enemy, and you need to get it out of your kid's life.

There are two things to know about cholesterol that are important for us nonscience heads: HDL and

LDL. HDL cholesterol levels are good, and LDLs are bad. If you want to know what they mean and all about the world of cholesterol, good. You just won't get it here, so search the Net. Remember, HDL = good, LDL = bad.

Olive oil, canola oil, and several others contain monounsaturated fats. They help raise HDLs, the good stuff. Peanut butter and salmon contain polyunsaturated fats. They also help with HDLs. Fats from animals, like butter and the yummy fat in a juicy ribeye, contain saturated fats. They raise the LDLs, the bad guys.

Trans fats raise the LDLs—no surprise there, right? But they also lower the HDLs! I told you they were bad. Some trans fats do occur naturally in some animals, but they aren't the same and aren't as dangerous at all. Trans fats are "necessary" because they extend the life of a product. The process that they go through keeps them from going rancid as fast, and may keep them in your body longer. So, the fats stay alive longer so you can die faster. Now do you see why I say to get rid of them?

You are going to be surprised when you see how many products contain trans fats. Read the ingredient labels no matter what the package says. The lovely FDA says that if a product contains less than a certain amount of trans fats, the company can label it trans-fat free. Sure, you can read that again if you like. But the ingredient list is where the clues are. If you see partially hydrogenated oil, the product has trans fats in it, even if it has been touted as having zero trans fats. It's a lie, plain and simple.

I know it's going to be tough to eliminate these fats, but just keep thinking about your kids and what's best for them. I believe that one day we will see trans fats banned in this country, but you should impose your own ban before that day happens.

~ 44 ~
Smile, give hugs, and love

– 44 –

Smile, give hugs, and love

*Every time you smile at someone, it is an action
of love, a gift to that person, a beautiful thing.*
                                                —Mother Teresa

You love your kids and obviously want what's best for them. As I have stated before, this book is about your approach toward healthy cooking and living. It is going to take work, time, and commitment to keep the lifestyle going, especially if your kids are in their teens already. Just remember that we as parents must do what's necessary to help them live happy and healthy lives.

This new life will be challenging, but don't forget to smile. It's hard to feel bad when you smile, so try it when you normally wouldn't. Life looks better, things seem easier, and even food tastes better when you smile.

Hugs can do great amounts of good—especially for children.
–Princess Diana

I know "Frankly, my dear, I don't give a [you-know-what]" is a pretty stern way to think, but the basis of what I'm talking about is absolutely necessary. We have to be parents when it comes to encouraging our kids to eat healthy. Just keep in mind that it shouldn't be a battle, because battles are the precursor to war. I am going to guess that when you had your children, you didn't declare war. When it comes to food choices, though, your kid will challenge you, and it may feel like a battle. But after all of the reading and the cooking and trying to help your kids eat well, hug your children, no matter what.

I don't mean to get all sappy on you, but I now want to bring together what I think is most important when it comes to things you should know about healthy cooking for kids: love your children in abundance.

If we truly love our kids, we won't feed them foods on a regular basis that are known to harm them. We shouldn't use garbage food as a sign of love. If we absolutely love our kids, we should take the time to find out how to get them to where we want them to be. I love my kiddies, and I know you love yours. Every day that you use love as your foundation, you've already completed 90 percent of your goal.

With love, I thank you and leave with a few beautiful quotes:

There is no sight on earth more appealing than the sight of a woman making dinner for someone she loves.

–Thomas Wolfe

Cooking is like love, it should be entered into with abandon or not at all.

–Harriet Van Horne

Cooking is at once child's play and adult joy. And cooking done with care is an act of love.

–Craig Claiborne

References

References

Chapter 12

"Frankly, my dear, I don't give a . . . !" –Rhett Butler, *Gone with the Wind*

Chapter 13

"Nobody puts Baby in a corner." –Johnny Castle, *Dirty Dancing*

Chapter 15

"Be the change you want to see in the world." –Mahatma Gandhi

Chapter 17

"Why, back in the 30s, children as young as five could work as they pleased; from textile factories to iron smelts. Yippee! Hurray!" –Mugatu, *Zoolander*

Chapter 24

"You can't show up at someone's house with Ring Dings and Pepsi!" –Elaine in "The Dinner Party," *Seinfeld*

Chapter 25
"I don't like potatoes but I love Tater Tots!" –Elijah Harper

Chapter 26
"Return to the root and you will find the meaning."–Sengstan

Chapter 28
"Constant dripping hollows out a stone." –Titus Lucretius Carus

Chapter 30
"Let there be work, bread, water, and salt for all." –Nelson Mandela

Chapter 31
"I'm going to make him an offer he can't refuse."
–Don Corleone, *The Godfather*

Chapter 40
"Never doubt that a small group of thoughtful, committed citizens can change the world; indeed, it's the only thing that ever has." –Margaret Mead

Check out these other books in the Good Things to Know series:

5 Things to Know for Successful and Lasting Weight Loss
(ISBN: 9781596525580, $9.99)
12 Things to Do to Quit Smoking
(ISBN: 9781596525849, $9.99)
Sorry For Your Loss: What People Who Are Grieving Wish You Knew
(ISBN: 9781596527478, $9.99)
20 Things To Know About Divorce
(ISBN: 9781596525993, $9.99)
21 Things To Create a Better Life
(ISBN: 9781596525269, $9.99)
24 Things You Can Do with Social Media to Help Get into College
(ISBN: 9781596527485, $9.99)
27 Things To Feng Shui Your Home
(ISBN: 9781596525672, $9.99)
27 Things To Know About Yoga
(ISBN: 9781596525900, $9.99)
29 Things To Know About Catholicism
(ISBN: 9781596525887, $9.99)
30 Things Future Dads Should Know About Pregnancy
(ISBN: 9781596525924, $9.99)
33 Things To Know About Raising Creative Kids
(ISBN: 9781596525627, $9.99)
34 Things To Know About Wine
(ISBN: 9781596525894, $9.99)
35 Things to Know to Raise Active Kids
(ISBN: 9781596525870, $9.99)
35 Things Your Teen Won't Tell You, So I Will
(ISBN: 9781596525542, $9.99)

Printed in the USA
CPSIA information can be obtained
at www.ICGtesting.com
JSHW052015140824
68134JS00027B/2485